Moving Pain Away RiVision®
An Innovative Physical Therapy Method

Moving Pain Away RiVision®
An Innovative Physical Therapy Method

Author
Rivi Belach Har-El PT PhD
Clinical Assistant Professor
State University of New York Downstate Medical Center
New York, USA

Foreword
Wen Ling PT PhD

Illustrator
Ziv Lenzner

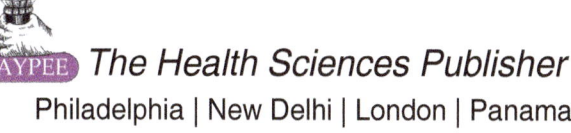

The Health Sciences Publisher
Philadelphia | New Delhi | London | Panama

Jaypee Brothers Medical Publishers (P) Ltd

Headquarters
Jaypee Brothers Medical Publishers (P) Ltd.
4838/24, Ansari Road, Daryaganj
New Delhi 110 002, India
Phone: +91-11-43574357
Fax: +91-11-43574314
E-mail: jaypee@jaypeebrothers.com

Overseas Offices

J.P. Medical Ltd.
83, Victoria Street, London
SW1H 0HW (UK)
Phone: +44-20 3170 8910
Fax: +44(0)20 3008 6180
E-mail: info@jpmedpub.com

Jaypee-Highlights Medical Publishers Inc.
City of Knowledge, Bld. 235, 2nd Floor, Clayton
Panama City, Panama
Phone: +1 507-301-0496
Fax: +1 507-301-0499
E-mail: cservice@jphmedical.com

Jaypee Medical Inc.
325 Chestnut Street
Suite 412
Philadelphia, PA 19106, USA
Phone: +1 267-519-9789
E-mail: support@jpmedus.com

Jaypee Brothers Medical Publishers (P) Ltd.
17/1-B, Babar Road, Block-B, Shaymali
Mohammadpur, Dhaka-1207
Bangladesh
Mobile: +08801912003485
E-mail: jaypeedhaka@gmail.com

Jaypee Brothers Medical Publishers (P) Ltd.
Bhotahity, Kathmandu, Nepal
Phone: +977-9741283608
E-mail: kathmandu@jaypeebrothers.com

Website: www.jaypeebrothers.com
Website: www.jaypeedigital.com

© 2017, Jaypee Brothers Medical Publishers

The views and opinions expressed in this book are solely those of the original contributor(s)/author(s) and do not necessarily represent those of editor(s) of the book.

All rights reserved. No part of this publication and may be reproduced, stored or transmitted in any form or by any means, electronic, mechanical, photocopying, recording or otherwise, without the prior permission in writing of the publishers.

All brand names and product names used in this book are trade names, service marks, trademarks or registered trademarks of their respective owners. The publisher is not associated with any product or vendor mentioned in this book.

Medical knowledge and practice change constantly. This book is designed to provide accurate, authoritative information about the subject matter in question. However, readers are advised to check the most current information available on procedures included and check information from the manufacturer of each product to be administered, to verify the recommended dose, formula, method and duration of administration, adverse effects and contraindications. It is the responsibility of the practitioner to take all appropriate safety precautions. Neither the publisher nor the author(s)/editor(s) assume any liability for any injury and/or damage to persons or property arising from or related to use of material in this book.

This book is sold on the understanding that the publisher is not engaged in providing professional medical services. If such advice or services are required, the services of a competent medical professional should be sought.

Every effort has been made where necessary to contact holders of copyright to obtain permission to reproduce copyright material. If any have been inadvertently overlooked, the publisher will be pleased to make the necessary arrangements at the first opportunity.

Inquiries for bulk sales may be solicited at: jaypee@jaypeebrothers.com

Moving Pain Away RiVision®: An Innovative Physical Therapy Method

First Edition: **2017**

ISBN: 978-93-86056-06-1

Printed at:

Dedication

In memory of my mom and dad, Hela and Hannan Belach; my grandparents, Rivka and Joshua Belach; and my in-laws, Helen and Ovadia Hardoon. Their heritage and life experience touched and influenced every aspect of my life.

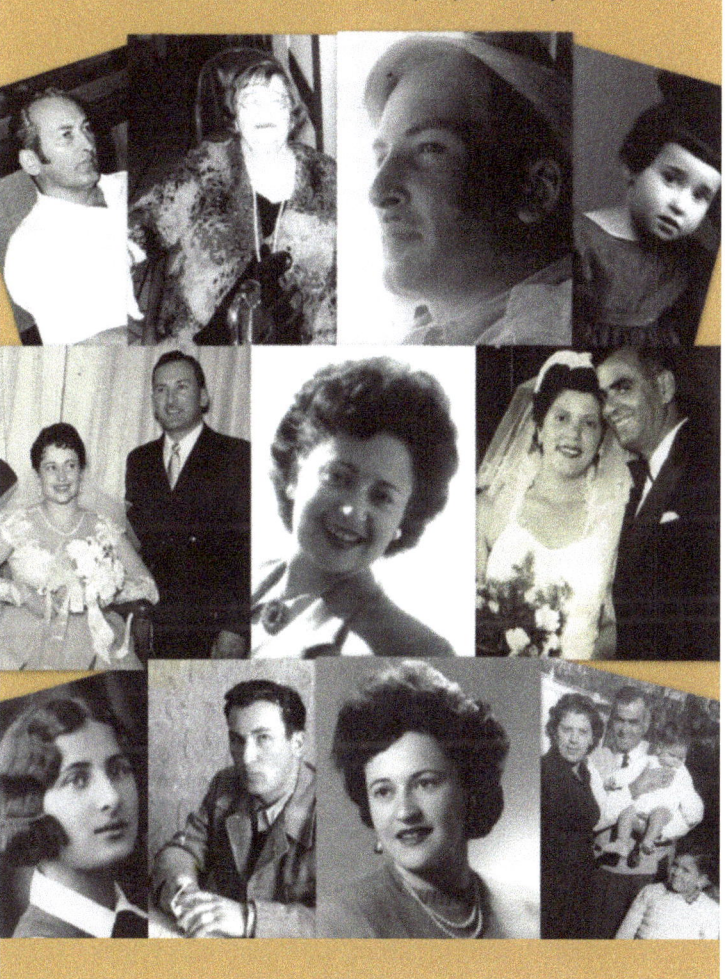

Foreword

As a physical therapist, I am often asked by friends and family members about pains and aches they are experiencing. The most common cause for pains and aches experienced is from the musculoskeletal system. If acute pain is not resolved, it becomes chronic pain. Chronic pain, defined as pain lasting for at least six months (Johannes et al., 2010), is a major health issue among adults in the United States. To investigate how frequently chronic pain occurs, Johannes and Associates (2010) sent a survey to 35,718 adults, representative of the United States adult population. The response rate of the internet-based survey was 75.7%, a relatively high response rate. About 41% of respondents reported having chronic, recurrent, or long-lasting pain (Johannes et al., 2010). The most common type of chronic pain was lower back pain, a type of musculoskeletal pain (Johannes et al., 2010). Findings from the Johannes study confirm my observation that many adults have chronic musculoskeletal pain and the need to find and to provide effective treatment for these patients.

However, there is little evidence on what type of treatment is most effective. For example, the Clinical Practice Guideline by the American College of Physicians and the American Pain Society for diagnosing and treating patients with chronic lower back pain included medications, interdisciplinary rehabilitation, exercise, acupuncture, massage, spinal manipulation, yoga, cognitive-behavioral therapy, and progressive relaxation (Chou et al., 2007). Part of the reason for a lack of clearly effective treatment is that physical, physiological, emotional, and psychological factors all impact the effectiveness of treatment. Thus, an effective treatment needs to address not just the physical and physiological issues, but also the psychological and emotional issues.

Dr. Rivi Belach Har-El is in a unique position as a physical therapist also trained in dance/movement therapy and guided imagery. She has incorporated all of her training to develop RiVision® to address the complex issues of patients with chronic musculoskeletal pain. The RiVision® approach presented in this book is based on her research and clinical experiences on patients with chronic musculoskeletal pain, not responding to traditional physical therapy interventions. Exercise, dance/movement therapy, and guided imagery are the three components of RiVision®. Each component can be delivered alone or with the other component(s).

Treatment principles and protocols identified in this book are appropriate for health professionals treating patients with chronic musculoskeletal pain. One unique aspect of the RiVision® method is listening to a patient's words describing his/her movement capability and primary movement patterns during the evaluation process (or changes in movement capability during the re-evaluation process). Four cases of typical patients with chronic musculoskeletal pain not responding to traditional treatment, presented in Chapter Five, walk readers through the complete process of RiVision®. The emotional aspect of each case reminds me that an effective treatment program needs to address physical, physiological, and emotional aspects of a patient. With guidance from a physical therapist, patients with chronic musculoskeletal pain can incorporate exercises published in this book.

Wen Ling PT PhD
Associate Professor
Department of Physical Therapy
New York University
New York, USA

References

1. Johannes CB, Le TK, Zhou X, Johnston JA, and Dworkin RH. The prevalence of chronic pain in the United States adults; Results of an internet-based survey. J Pain 11(11): 1230-1239, 2010.
2. Chou R, Qaseem A, Snow V, Casey D, Cross T, Shekelle P, and Owens DK. Diagnosis and treatment of low back pain; A joint clinical practice guideline from the American College of Physicians and the American Pain Society. Ann Int Med 147(7):478-491, 2007.

Preface

Chronic pain is not merely a physical sensation resulting from a physical injury. It is a multifaceted experience influenced by many factors, among which are depression, anger, and anxiety. Although physical therapy does provide psychological benefits, it does not address subconscious processes, like mindfulness-based techniques do. Unlike other physical therapy treatments that deal with chronic physical pain and musculoskeletal disorders, RiVision® simultaneously relates to a large array of physical and emotional manifestations of pain.

Patients and therapists practicing this method are encouraged to develop a greater awareness of their body-mind weaknesses at an early stage of the treatment by identifying the "Repetitive Stress Pattern" that may have led to their chronic pain.

RiVision® consists of elements, such as physical therapy, dance/movement therapy, and guided imagery practice. In physical therapy, we relate to the patient's range of motion, pain level, posture, and function level. Dance/movement therapy addresses the patient's use of vertical, horizontal and sagittal planes of motion as well as the general typical pattern of movement. In guided imagery, RiVision® relates to the images the person perceives and describes inside and outside his/her body in relation to daily encounters with other people and events.

The art of integrating various modalities within RiVision® in a way that will best fit the patient's needs is of great importance. To accomplish the desired outcome, it is recommended that the treatment method be specifically tailored to each patient by following one of the seven protocols of treatment outlined in this book.

Rivi Belach Har-El

Acknowledgments

The completion of my book would not have been possible without continual professional, academic and emotional support from family, friends, patients and professional colleagues. A special thanks to Mr. Ziv Lenzner for portraying with accuracy, sensitivity and unique understanding of the human body via his illustrations; to Elite Ben-Yosef, PhD for helping with editing while figuring out the depth of the method behind the written word; and to Professor Mary Clare Lennon's professional support and friendship.

I was very fortunate to have Professor Sherri Weiser as a supportive, sensitive and encouraging advisor. Special thanks to Dr. Catherine Shainberg, who taught me guided imagery and helped with its incorporation into my treatment philosophy.

Finally, my very special warm gratitude and love to my closest family. I thank my husband, Professor Gady Har-El, and my sons Amir and Ilan, for their unconditional support and love. Gady and Ilan sacrificed their valuable time and energy to edit and comment on my work.

About the Author

Dr. Rivi Belach Har-El has over 33 years of experience in treating chronic pain and musculoskeletal disorders. In 2000, Dr. Rivi received her PhD in Physical Therapy from New York University, New York, USA.

Throughout her career, she enhanced her knowledge of pain in all its manifestations by studying psychology and dance/movement therapy, and by exposing herself to various integrated forms of chronic pain treatment. She came to understand that health caregivers need to be able to relate a patient's symptoms to what is happening simultaneously in their body and mind. This realization led her to develop the RiVision® method.

She is a Clinical Assistant Professor at the State University of New York Downstate Medical Center, New York, USA, where she teaches future therapists how to utilize body-mind awareness and the RiVision® method.

Dr. Rivi is the founder of the RiVision® Healing Center in New York.

About the Illustrator

Ziv Lenzner is an Israeli painter and a lecturer of academic drawing, concept art, anatomical and realistic painting for the Department of Animation and Arts of Minshar Art Academy in Tel Aviv, Israel. He specializes in painting and drawing anatomy. Ziv has also taught drawing and oil painting at the Israel Museum in Jerusalem and the Morasha Jerusalem College of Arts in Jerusalem.

Contents

1. **Introduction: The Roots of the RiVision® Method** 1
2. **The Need to Observe the "Entire Body Manifestation/ Movement" When Treating Chronic Pain** 7
3. **The Components of RiVision®: Physical Therapy, Dance/Movement Therapy and Guided Imagery** 11
   - Physical Therapy (PT) *11*
   - Dance/Movement Therapy (DMT) *13*
   - Guided Imagery *14*
4. **The Basic Principles of RiVision®** 17
   - Guidelines: Tailoring RiVision® to the Patient *18*
   - Five Motion Factors of RiVision® *20*
   - Awareness *21*
   - Grounding *33*
   - Pacing *40*
   - Orienting *46*
   - Muscle Tension *51*
5. **Case Studies: Treatment Goals, Exercises and Outcomes** 61
   - Case Study # 1—Betty *61*
   - Case Study # 2—Wen *86*
   - Case Study # 3—Cha *103*
   - Case Study # 4—Jane *123*
   - Summary *135*

6. **Apply the RiVision® Method** — 137
   - Finding the "Repetitive Stress Pattern" *137*
   - Charting your Responses *138*
   - Analyzing the Patient's Responses *141*
   - How to Utilize RiVision® *141*

7. **Summary** — 145

Bibliography — 149

Appendix — 151

Index — 165

CHAPTER 1

Introduction: The Roots of the RiVision® Method

This book explores the benefits of RiVision®, an innovative physical therapy method that is designed to treat musculoskeletal injuries and chronic pain. This method uniquely combines physical therapy, dance/movement therapy (DMT) and guided imagery so that, working together, they can be more effective than they would be if used separately. The RiVision® method stands for one's ability to envision her body differently; to see, identify and revise the way she relates to and treats her chronic pain.

In 2000, I completed my doctoral dissertation from the New York University Physical Therapy Department, where I examined a new treatment intervention for people with chronic neck pain. My work was to compare neck exercises combined with either dance/movement therapy (DMT—a form of intervention that uses dance as a process which furthers the emotional and physical integration of the individual) or with aerobic training (AT). Treatment outcome in each group was measured by the effect on mood state, pain perception and cervical range of motion (CROM).

My findings indicated that DMT was as effective in improving mood state, decreasing pain perception, and increasing CROM as AT. In addition, it is postulated that in DMT, the spontaneous, pleasurable expenditure of energy offers relaxation and the sublimation of worries (Payne, 1992). The effects of DMT on mood can be explained by the theory of catharsis and spontaneous expression through movement. Leste and Rust (1984) theorized that the cathartic nature of dance, with its concomitant emotional expression, release of tension, anger or frustration, can alter the individual's mood state. Therefore, DMT has the potential to offer greater benefits than AT.

In my practice I incorporate guided imagery exercises that have been shown to be effective for patients with pain conditions, such as imagining a healing light. My study results, along with 33 years of experience treating patients with various musculoskeletal disorders and chronic pain, led me to develop and implement RiVision®, which combines physical therapy, DMT and guided imagery.

Chronic pain is not merely a physical sensation resulting from a physical injury; it is a multifaceted experience influenced by emotional factors, such as depression, stress, anger and anxiety. The use of physical therapy and psychological services is common practice in these cases. In 1983, after graduating from physical therapy school, I often observed that patients needed to express their emotions while receiving conventional physical therapy treatment. The patients would lie on the treatment bed letting out a wide array of feelings, including negative personal experiences from their lives.

At first I was reluctant to respond to these emotions since I was not equipped with the appropriate educational background. As time progressed I realized that I needed to enhance my knowledge of pain in all its manifestations by studying psychology and exposing myself to various integrated forms of therapy related to chronic pain. Recognizing the influences affecting those with chronic pain, I have come to understand that health caregivers need to be able to relate a patient's symptoms to what is happening simultaneously in their body and mind. I learned that DMT and guided imagery are the best ways to address a patient's psychological presentation, which often manifested in their posture, gestures and movements.

My training began with a Bachelor of Physical Therapy (BPT) degree, followed by a Master of Science (MS) degree in DMT. The latter is a form of intervention that uses dance/movement rather than words/talking as the main mode of treatment to facilitate the emotional and physical integration of the individual.

It was my intention to incorporate the knowledge and experience I acquired in these professional preparation programs, along with my training in guided imagery, to further benefit those patients who sought help due to various musculoskeletal disorders such as lower back pain. However, for many years I was puzzled by just how to integrate these different yet complementary therapies. I wanted to be able to look at an individual through a broader spectrum than one that is used in or as independent physical entities, but as entities connected to an individual's emotional issues. The idea is that behind the painful, injured body parts there is a human being with an untold story. Pain can be the body's way of expressing that story.

In cases where the traditional physical therapy approach does not suffice for alleviating pain, we must look for other treatment solutions for the complex and mysterious ways a body cries for help. Despite the idea that there are psychological benefits to physical therapeutic exercises, conventional therapy typically does not address the subconscious processes involved in chronic pain. In my work, I have found that the simultaneous usage of physical exercises and modalities relating to the subconscious is superior to the usage of physical interventions alone.

During my training in DMT, I studied the work of Warren Lamb, whose work influenced my final thesis titled, *The Psychological Implications of Moving in Different Planes* (Har-El, 1991). In my thesis I explored the relationships between body movement style and three personality traits: (1) risk-taking, (2) level of self-esteem and (3) social participation. An analysis of the test results from a group of DMT students supported a correlation between an individual's movement pattern and certain personality traits. The main findings were:

- People who move their body back and forth (the sagittal plane) more often than up and down or side-to-side (vertical and horizontal planes) are more likely to have a higher score in risk-taking than in self-esteem and social participation.
- People who use up and down motions (vertical plane) more often than the back and forth and side-to-side motions (sagittal and horizontal planes) are more likely to have a higher score in self-esteem than in risk-taking and social participation.

These findings imply that there is a relationship between the way people move their bodies and their state of mind or well-being. Patients may develop body misalignment, pain and discomfort for various reasons. When they seek help from a physical therapist they expect to receive traditional therapy involving physical modalities such as massage and therapeutic exercises to treat the injured area.

However, when I observed my patients' movement patterns and postures it became obvious to me that I should consider their movement behavior and general well-being as part of their treatment as well as their physical complaint. I realized, based on my patients' personal verbal and nonverbal communication with me, that the patients' movement patterns/movement characteristics could reveal further information leading to the source of the pain.

The material presented to you is a culmination of this research supported by 33 years of practice and my PhD dissertation. In this book, I introduce the RiVision® method (Chapter 1) followed by the need to observe the entire body manifestation and movement (Chapter 2). I explain the three components of RiVision® (Chapter 3): (1) physical therapy, (2) DMT and (3) guided imagery. Then I discuss the seven treatment protocols used in RiVision® (Chapter 4) and the five underlying principles (motion factors)—awareness, grounding, pacing, orienting and muscle tension—using several principles of the Action Profiling theory (for further details *see* Appendix).

This section is followed by four case studies detailing the stories and treatment paths of four patients (Chapter 5). Each patient's treatment includes the treatment goal and the exercises tailored to achieve that goal. These stories show how RiVision® helped one patient to overcome chronic physical and emotional pain, and learn how to respect and love oneself. You will learn about another patient who suffered from asthma while her body posture was concaved, as if to protect herself. With therapy she was able to open up her movement (erect her body and open her chest), which led to her gradual opening up emotionally. She was also able to use her inhaler less frequently, and her posture and upper body flexibility improved significantly. I also show how a man in a stressful and demanding profession, that manifested in chronic neck pain and rigidity, was eventually able to move his entire upper body and neck without pain as a result of the use of imagery and physical movement. Lastly, another story shows how someone extremely frail can develop her self-esteem and inner strength, and learn to protect herself and her body so that she is able to face life with greater stamina and endurance.

In Chapter 6, I explain how to apply the RiVision® method by finding the reader's "Repetitive Stress Pattern" (RSP) and analyzing it. Last is a summary and conclusion (Chapter 7). In the Appendix, I include more technical details geared toward the practitioner.

This book is for chronic pain sufferers who have not been completely helped by traditional therapies. RiVision® offers a thorough treatment approach that is not a quick fix, but rather a comprehensive approach to a long lasting condition. The purpose of this book is to familiarize you, the reader, with the core principles of RiVision®. The RiVision® principles presented in this book may also enrich practitioners who are interested in learning about an innovative treatment for their patients. RiVision® offers both patients and practitioners a method for overcoming pain by uniquely combining physical therapy, DMT and guided imagery.

CHAPTER 2

The Need to Observe the "Entire Body Manifestation/Movement" When Treating Chronic Pain

Patients may develop body misalignment, pain and discomfort for various reasons. Through musculoskeletal and biomechanical responses the body holds emotional issues in its muscles and bones. The muscle tension theory, which attempts to explain why mood and pain frequently coexist, suggests that anxiety, which is frequently associated with depression, can elicit increased muscle tension (Chapman, 1990). Tightness and spasm of the soft tissue following pain or trauma lead to a decrease in muscle activity and reduce the range of motion, according to Porterfield and DeRosa (1995).

Muscle tension not only affects musculoskeletal conditions, but may also exacerbate other diseases, such as asthma. Musculoskeletal dysfunction and pain were found in adults with asthma according to Lunardi et al. (2011). The mechanical alterations related to the overload of respiratory muscles observed in adults with persistent asthma might lead to the development of chronic alterations in posture, musculoskeletal dysfunction and pain.

A useful framework is described by Lamb (1981). He offers a movement observation method that emphasizes the relationship between posture-gesture-mergers, personality traits and motivation: "It has been found that everyone has a distinctive pattern of integrated movement which endures throughout life. When observed and matched against a framework, it has come to be known as an Action-Profile," (Lamb, 1981, p. 21). The Action-Profile is an observation method used for studying managerial and work behavior via movements aiming to enhance personal performance and team organizational effectiveness.

The Action-Profile assessment is based upon detailed observation of minute variations in nonverbal behavior, specifically movements. The analysis is concerned with what happens between positions. For example, how the arms and legs make the transition from uncrossed/unfolded to crossed/folded. Is the transition being executed with a firm, light, abrupt, cautious, or direct movement quality? The particular quality of the movement indicates that the individual is expending a particular type of energy. For example, "a directing movement indicates the cultivation of focused energy," which generates "investigatory thinking such as probing for information and making distinctions" (Ramsden & Zachrias, 1993). The part of RiVision® that deals with dance/movement therapy (DMT) is derived from four motion factors used by the Action-Profile and will be detailed in Chapter 4 (Weight, Time, Pace and Flow). For more details about the Action-Profile, see Appendix.

Influenced by Action-Profile, I developed a unique approach of analyzing human motion, which I then used to enhance my patients' performance. My patients were referred to physical therapy with complaints of musculoskeletal disorders including neck and back pain. However, my goal was different from an "Action-Profile" consultant. I focused on the characteristic pattern of movement that may have caused their misalignment, dysfunction or pain. More specifically, I related to Moore's (1982) three planes of motion: (1) vertical, (2) sagittal and (3) horizontal. These three planes intersect at the center of the body in different directions (Fig. 2.1):

1. *The door plane* (representing the vertical plane of motion) slices vertically through the body from head to toe, separating the front of the body from the back. The door plane's primary dimension is height; its secondary dimension is width. It extends up and down and to the right and left of the body.

2. *The wheel plane* (representing the sagittal plane of motion) bisects the body along its vertical axis, separating the right side from the left side. Its primary dimension is depth; its secondary dimension is height. It extends in front of and behind the body, and also upward and downward.

3. *The table plane* (representing the horizontal plane of motion) bisects the body at the waist level. Its primary dimension is width; its secondary dimension is depth. It extends to the right and left and in front of and behind the body. It separates the head, chest and arms from the hips and legs (Moore, 1982, p. 69).

The Need to Observe the "Entire Body Manifestation/Movement" 9

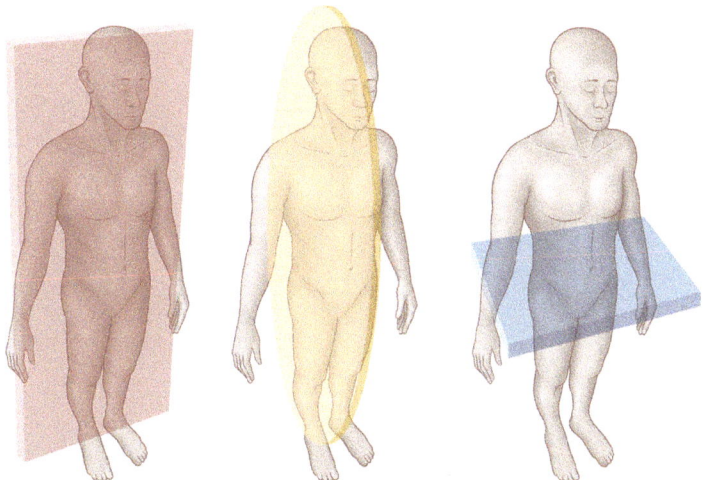

Fig. 2.1: Three planes of motion: Vertical (door), sagittal (wheel), and horizontal (table).

I was interested in finding, for example, what happens to a person who utilizes the up and down spine motion (vertical plane of motion) more than the side-to-side spine motion (horizontal plane of motion). How will that person experience her body compared to someone who utilizes the side-to-side spine motion more than the up and down spine motion? Will the tension in the musculature of the back be distributed differently in the three individuals? Will posture be affected by the difference in spine motion and body mechanics? Why would she prefer to use an up and down motion compared to a side-to-side or back and forth motion? Is she conscious of her movement pattern, and if so, to what degree?

In order to thoroughly evaluate and analyze the complexity of the body disorder/discomfort, I drew from the following elements within physical therapy, DMT, and guided imagery practice. In physical therapy, I related to the patient's range of motion, pain level, posture and function levels. In DMT, I related to the patient's usage of the vertical, horizontal and sagittal planes of motion as well as the general typical pattern of movement. In guided imagery, I related to the images the person described inside and outside her body in relationship to daily encounters with other people and events.

Chapter 3

The Components of RiVision®: Physical Therapy, Dance/Movement Therapy and Guided Imagery

PHYSICAL THERAPY (PT)

Hands-On Techniques

Manual/hands-on therapy is defined as a clinical approach utilizing skilled, specific hands-on techniques, including but not limited to manipulation/mobilization used by the physical therapist to diagnose and treat soft tissues and joint structures. These techniques are used for modulating pain, increasing range of motion (ROM), reducing or eliminating soft tissue inflammation, inducing relaxation, improving tissue repair, extensibility, and stability, facilitating movement and improving function.

Manual/hands-on techniques that I found to be the most helpful to my patients and therefore I employ are: joint mobilization, soft tissue mobilization, myofascial release and body-tuning.

A. *Joint mobilization* involves painless loosening up of the restricted joint and increasing its mobility by providing slow speed and increasing range of movement directed at the actual bone surface.

B. *Soft tissue mobilization* consists of rhythmic stretching and moderate pressure to break up inelastic or fibrous muscle tissue. The procedure is usually applied to musculature surrounding the spine and is done in various intensities based on the patient's needs.

C. *Myofascial release* is a connective tissue technique that combines fascial elongation with varying amounts of stretching.

D. *Body tuning*, developed by Dr. Shmuel Tatz, crosses modalities of many techniques combining Western and Eastern practices and emphasizing hands-on work on multiple joints related to the disorder. For example, elbow pain treatment includes treatment of the entire arm and upper body.

Therapeutic Exercises

Therapeutic exercises, commonly used in physical therapy, place stresses and forces on the body systems in a progressive fashion in order to develop, improve, restore or maintain normal function through the development of strength, endurance, flexibility, relaxation and coordination.

Functional Approaches

Functional approaches concentrate on educating one's neuromuscular or sensory-motor system to expand the range of one's movements, thus affecting how one functions (Knaster, 1996). These include, among others, the Alexander and Feldenkrais techniques.

A. *Alexander technique* is a method that works to change (movement) habits in everyday activities. It is a simple and practical method for improving ease and freedom of movement, balance, support and coordination. The technique teaches the appropriate amount of effort and use for a particular activity. It is not a series of treatments or exercises, but rather a reeducation of the mind and body (Andrade and Clifford, 2008).

B. *Feldenkrais technique* focuses on replacing old habits of movement with new, healthier ones. It comprises a set of exercises that focus on slow, non-aerobic movement with minimum effort and maximum efficiency (Feldenkrais, 1990).

Breathing Exercises

In addition to the hands-on techniques, therapeutic exercises and functional approaches (mentioned above), I incorporate breathing exercises into many of the treatment protocols. Breathing exercises influence the rate, depth and distribution of ventilation or the muscular activity associated with breathing (Scully and Barnes, 1989). It is a simple, yet powerful relaxation technique. It is easy to learn and provides a quick way of decreasing stress levels.

DANCE/MOVEMENT THERAPY (DMT)

Dance/movement therapy (DMT) is a form of intervention that uses dance and movement as a process which furthers the emotional and physical integration of the individual. According to the Dance Therapy Association, DMT involves the psychotherapeutic use of movement to further the emotional, cognitive, physical and social integration of the individual (www.adta.org/about_dmt).

A basic premise underlying DMT practice is that there is no division between mind and body behavior. Body movements reflect emotional states, and changes in movement behavior can lead to changes in the psyche (Knaster, 1996; Levy, 1988). Therapy starts at the patient's current physical and emotional level and allows for change and growth through the expansion of movement and extension of self (Schmais, 1974).

The effect of DMT on mood can be explained by the theory of catharsis and spontaneous expression through movement. Leste and Rust (1984) theorized that the cathartic nature of dance, with its concomitant emotional expression, and release of tension, anger or frustration, can alter the individual's mood state. It is postulated that in DMT, the spontaneous, pleasurable expenditure of energy offers relaxation and sublimation of worries (Payne, 1992). The trust established between the patient and the therapist during the session leads to an openness, which allows patients to express themselves physically and emotionally (Kruas, Hilsendager and Dixon, 1991).

The Chace Technique

The theoretical foundation of dance therapy was laid down by six major pioneers; among them Marian Chace (Levy, 1988) on whose work my treatment is based. This technique utilizes dance as the primary mode of interaction, communication and expression. The Chace technique focuses on body action, symbolism, the therapeutic movement relationship, and the group of patients' rhythmic movement relationship.

Through *bodily action*, the patients gain mobility and an enhanced awareness of how, when, and where they move various body parts. Changes in body action produce changes in emotional states, and emotional states may be recognized through breathing patterns and muscular tension. For example, when encountering a patient who seems to be physically and emotionally rigid, the therapist may use bodily actions (such as spreading motions or relaxation exercises that break the musculature rigidity) to unblock the tension stored in the body. The therapist will introduce motions that can develop the patient's readiness for emotional responsiveness and unblock physical restrictions.

Symbolism in DMT provides a medium by which a patient can recall and reenact repressed experiences that are associated with negative thoughts, emotions, and maladaptive movements. Symbolism may represent an object, a person, a feeling or an idea. For example, a negative personal feeling can express itself through aggressive motions, such as punching. In this case, the punching motion acts as a symbol for the negative personal feeling (Sandel, 1993).

The third theoretical concept—*therapeutic movement relationship*—relates to the nonverbal and symbolic communications through dance between the therapist and patient. This interaction occurs through the therapist's mirroring of the individual's specific movement pattern, then expanding and clarifying the meaning behind it (Levy, 1988). The interaction can highlight to the patient that, for instance, she is stuck in her chest movement. She only moves her chest back and forth. She then will be encouraged to expand her chest motion by moving it up and down and from side-to-side, leading to an expansion in both herself and her motions.

The rhythmic movement relationship, the fourth theoretical concept in Chace's work, relates to the power of group rhythm action as expression of emotions and feelings in an organized, repetitive, and harmonious manner. A group of patients will be encouraged to move in synchrony, using rhythm to organize the expression of thoughts and feelings into meaningful dance action. For example, the group "frustration issue" will be directed in motion to an execution of a sharp, straightforward intense motion done by all patients together while providing a group structure and a supportive environment.

GUIDED IMAGERY

Images are thoughts that draw on our senses. They may involve one, several, or all the following senses: hearing, taste, movement, vision, touch, smell and inner sensation. The goal of guided imagery is to make beneficial physical changes in the body by repeatedly visualizing the sensations associated with the experience. An example of a guided imagery exercise to mop up an inflammation is:

> "Breathe out three times. Imagine that with a pure white cotton wad you mop up the red inflamed wet color until it permeates the cotton. Then take the cotton and throw it over your left shoulder. There, it is gone! When you look again, the area of your pain looks clean and light. The pain is gone. Breathe out and open your eyes" (Shainberg, 2005, p. 98).

An image, like any other thought, sparks an electrical chain of events in the brain. For example, imagery influences endorphin secretions which then affect a person's mood.

The therapist will guide the patient in the process of visualization to help them "*see in*" pictures. Dr. Shainberg (2005, p. 98) gives an exercise illustrating how to see a physical, emotional and mental pain:

> "Close your eyes. Breathe out three times, counting from three to one, seeing the numbers clearly. See the number one as being tall, clear, very straight and very bright. Now become aware of a pain in your body. It can be a physical, emotional or mental pain. Just locate its place in your body. Then imagine turning your eyes inward and traveling down to the source of your pain. 'See' it with your inner eye. How does it appear to you? What color is it? Does it smell? Does it have a texture? Is it hot or cold, inflamed or dull, wet or dry? Describe everything you 'see' about your pain. In 'seeing' it, you become true to its source."

Wright and Mischel (1982) used a modified version of the Mood Adjective Check List and found that imagery alters emotional states. Imagery of happy events led to positive feelings and imagery of sad events led to negative feelings.

In the next chapter, I present the guidelines to RiVision® and examine the five motion factors derived from Action-Profiling and modified for RiVision® (for more on Action-Profiling, *see* Appendix). The patient is evaluated, treated, and then re-evaluated to determine the progress and course of treatment to follow.

CHAPTER 4

The Basic Principles of RiVision®

RiVision® incorporates a succession of questions and answers between the therapist and the patient regarding feelings and sensations. The process flow is based on patient responses. I therefore consider it of great importance to present to the reader the sequence of questions and answers between the therapist and the patient, which is used to facilitate the treatment incorporating the motion factors.

One part of the underlying principles of RiVision® is to achieve greater range of expansion within the patient's movement patterns. An example of expansion of motion leading to a more balanced usage of the movements would be a patient who learns to extend her spine and movements upward, and open herself up to the world after years of moving her spine downward and being closed off to the world. Oftentimes, restriction of spine motion and body movements implies being defensive and protective, while opening up and expanding imply emotional openness and greater confidence.

By attaining a greater expansion of body motion, a patient would be capable of assuming a more balanced use of motion factors: (1) grounding, (2) pacing, (3) orienting and (4) muscle tension. A patient will also be able to assume a more balanced use of the three planes of movement: (1) vertical, (2) sagittal and (3) horizontal (Fig. 4.1).

The art of integrating various modalities, incorporated within RiVision®, that will best fit the patient's needs is a complex one. The treatment method is specifically tailored to each patient. RiVision® gradually identifies the appropriate mode of therapy as the treatment progresses, without a predetermined protocol. It is based on the therapist's and patient's continuous communication. Some patients may be open to practice part or the full range of RiVision® modalities,

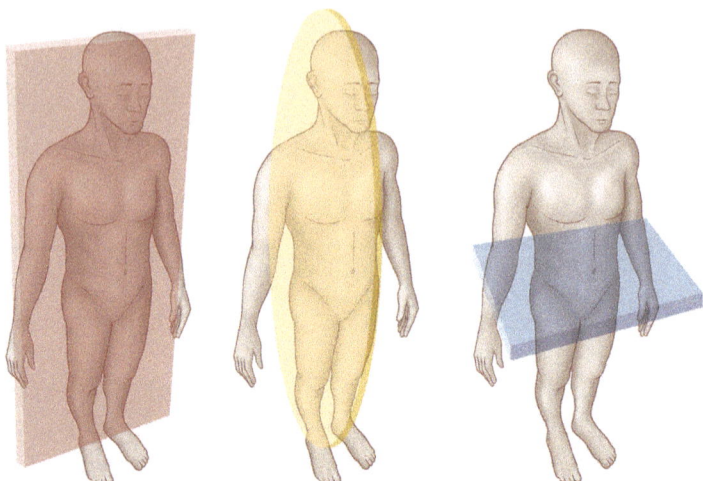

Fig. 4.1: Three planes of motion: Vertical (door), sagittal (wheel), and horizontal (table).

while others may be reluctant to do so. Without patient openness and belief in the possibilities this process holds, change and success cannot occur.

GUIDELINES: TAILORING RIVISION® TO THE PATIENT

There are seven protocols that are used in RiVision® (*see* description of the RiVision® components in Chapter 3).

The Seven Treatment Protocols

The single therapies:
1. Physical therapy
2. Dance/movement therapy (DMT)
3. Guided imagery

The combined therapies:
4. Combination of physical therapy and DMT
5. Combination of physical therapy and guided imagery
6. Combination of DMT and guided imagery
7. Combination of physical therapy, DMT and guided imagery

The following are practical guidelines for the entire process of the initial evaluation, modality selection, use of RiVision®, feedback with re-evaluation, and disposition with home program regimen and self-assessment.

A. The therapist evaluates the patient using conventional physical therapy methods. Initial evaluation includes subjective complaints, objective physical findings, assessment and plan of treatment. The therapist listens to the patient's life story as it is related to her chronic pain/discomfort. The information gathered during the course of the evaluation relates to the physical, social and emotional states of the patient. In most cases, the therapist will begin with physical therapy only. It is common to see that as the patient's therapy advances, she feels more comfortable opening up about personal issues as they may be related to her physical and emotional pain.

B. The therapist and the patient determine how to proceed by selecting one of the seven RiVision®'s protocols mentioned above.

C. The patient is treated for four weeks and re-evaluated to determine whether to continue or change the treatment option. For example, a patient is treated with physical therapy alone during the first four weeks. The treatment appears to be helpful but limited. She is able to stretch her arms further up (greater range of motion and flexibility) than before but inside she feels extremely vulnerable and needs to protect herself by returning to a low curved position, keeping her arms closer to her chest for security. The patient and therapist feel that the use of physical therapy and DMT while she expresses her emotions will bring a faster recovery.

D. Verbal and nonverbal interactions and communication between therapist and patient are significant factors determining treatment benefits to the patient. A significant part of the evaluation and re-evaluation relies on subjective descriptions such as, "I feel more secure to erect my upper back and neck" or "My back is heavy from carrying family issues."

E. Re-evaluation of patient progress occurs every four weeks. It is common to find in RiVision® that combined therapies (protocols 4 to 7) are used more often than single therapies (protocols 1 to 3).

F. The home program regimen is designed to include therapeutic exercises and guided imagery. The patient uses a notebook

Table 4.1: Event/Interaction-Feelings-Sensations		
Event/Interaction	Feelings	Sensations

to chart in great detail what was prescribed to her and what was eventually achieved during and after the therapy session. In addition, she will fill out Table 4.1 describing the feelings (sad, happy, etc.) and the physical sensations (numb, cold, etc.) brought about by an event or interaction occurring in her daily life and how they affected her musculoskeletal system.

G. The patient's progress is evaluated based on, among other factors, the feedback on the execution of the exercises, her feelings, and her sensations related to daily life activities. Examples of the intricate stage-by-stage development of the treatment have been explored in this book.

After completing the reading of this book, you will have a greater understanding of the RiVision® method. You may be able to use some parts of the method independently or you may need to seek help from practitioners who are trained in one of the treatment modalities: physical therapy, DMT or guided imagery.

After you become familiar with the physical therapy, DMT, and guided imagery components of RiVision® (Chapter 3) and the treatment protocols offered, I will examine the five motion factors derived from Action Profiling and modified for RiVision® (for more on Action Profiling *see* Appendix).

FIVE MOTION FACTORS OF RIVISION®

Awareness, grounding, pacing, orienting and muscle tension in relation to both the physical and the emotional aspects of being.

Awareness

As it relates to RiVision®, awareness refers to how conscious the patient is of her feelings, the sense of her body, and the space around her. Feelings are emotions such as sadness or joy. Sensing relates to the experience in the body, such as tightness or tingling.

The groundwork for RiVision® is facilitated by using exercises that heighten the patient's *awareness*. For example, when relating to the sensation in her tight front chest area, can she also relate to the emotion that she may be experiencing in the same area? Is she oblivious to her sensations and feelings in the front of her chest? *Note*: these exercises are not given in any specific order since they come up in the context of interaction.

The following is a series of exercises that I commonly use to assist those patients who are not fully aware of their breathing patterns, parts of their body or their entire body and their feelings. For each exercise, I have given you an example of a patient's response. In practice, the responses may vary in nature and also change as the patient moves forward in her therapy. These examples are intended to help you understand the flow of the therapy. You are encouraged to try the exercises and write down your responses relating to the event, the way you felt and how you sensed your body (Table 4.1).

AWARENESS EXERCISE 1

Evaluate your breathing pattern when you move and do not move. Where do you breathe from (nose or mouth) and to (your front, side or back of the chest or your abdominal cavity)? How much do you expand your chest and in which direction? Is your breath shallow or deep? Do you feel that you use your lungs to fully expand while breathing?

Patient's response:

"I cannot breathe deeply. Something stands in my way. I feel that the expansion in my chest occurs only in the front part of my chest. I am not aware of any side or back movements."

Reader's response:

_____
_____
_____
_____
_____
_____
_____
_____
_____
_____
_____
_____
_____
_____
_____
_____
_____

AWARENESS EXERCISE 2

> *Feel your feet and check if the muscles in your feet are relaxed. If you are not aware of your feet, allow yourself to contract and release the foot muscles 10–15 times until you have a greater awareness of them. Then move slowly up the body to your shins, thighs and pelvis, as you continue performing the same exercise of activating the muscles. If you are aware of your leg muscles now, check if they are relaxed. If the feeling is not there yet, continue with the contracting and releasing exercises.*

Patient's response:
"After the contracting and releasing exercises, my lower body, from my hips down, was very relaxed, but my upper body is sensing constant, moderate tension, particularly at the shoulders and the neck."

Reader's response:

AWARENESS EXERCISE 3

> *When relating to the horizontal, vertical and sagittal planes of movement, what is your dominant movement style? To use the horizontal plane, move your torso and extremities from side-to-side. To use the vertical plane, move your torso and extremities up and down. To use the sagittal plane, move your torso and extremities back and forth. Do you have a particular plane that you use more dominantly than others or not (see Fig. 4.1)?*

Patient's response:
"I am using the vertical plane of moving my torso upright in most motions, more than other dimensions of motion. I am not clear why, but this is my way."

Reader's response:

AWARENESS EXERCISE 4

> *Where do you initiate your movements from when you are interacting with others and walking around? Is it from your chest, hands, wrists, shoulders or head? For example, when you initiate a conversation, are you primarily moving your hands more than your chest? Are you using the right arm more than the left? Does your chest move while conversing? Try to recall different instances in which you are engaged using your torso and extremities. See yourself like an actor/actress on a stage—how do you talk, move, and engage?*

Patient's response:
"During my conversations, I feel that I breathe shallowly while my fingers and hands move like an acrobat in all directions. My shoulders and upper body are stagnant, in general. When I am walking, I tend to move my upper extremities a great deal by swinging my arms back and forth while minimally moving the torso and chest."

Reader's response:
_____
_____
_____
_____
_____
_____
_____
_____
_____
_____
_____
_____
_____
_____
_____
_____
_____

AWARENESS EXERCISE 5

Once you are familiar with your inherent movement patterns, do you think you would be able to expand upon them while interacting with others? For instance, instead of using your arms only in back and forth directions, expand your repertoire to move them from side-to-side and up and down as well.

Imagine that you are an actor on the stage and you are broadening your repertoire. Practice doing so using imagery: close your eyes, breathe out three times and see yourself in the middle of a meadow. The temperature is pleasant, you are relaxed and calm. See yourself walking in the meadow swinging your arms in all directions, being very free and agile. Were you able to imagine yourself moving slightly differently from the way you are used to or not? Check your movement style in relation to the usage of the horizontal, sagittal and vertical planes.

Patient's response:
"I was not able to use my arms differently. Nothing changed with the way I walk. However, I felt freer in the torso region and my breathing was deeper than before."

Reader's response:
_____
_____
_____
_____
_____
_____
_____
_____
_____
_____
_____

AWARENESS EXERCISE 6

> *Move freely and let your arms move in different directions. Enjoy the freedom of the dance and see if your movement style is altered somehow. Try to define your pattern of movement based on the horizontal, vertical and sagittal planes.*

Patient's response:
"I was surprised that I was able to move my arms in different directions without a great deal of effort. It was easy to execute while I was aware of my torso and chest, which were moving from side-to-side and rotating more than I had ever done before."

Reader's response:

_____
_____
_____
_____
_____
_____
_____
_____
_____
_____
_____
_____
_____
_____
_____
_____

AWARENESS EXERCISE 7

> *How often do you repeat your inherent movement pattern in daily life? Do you use your fingers and hands all of the time (90-100%), or less often (about 80-89%, or 60-79%, or 40-59%, or 20-39%, or 0-19% of the time) when interacting with others? Are you able to change your inherent movement pattern at times? Has the percentage use of your inherent movement pattern changed since you began treatment? Are you able to move your torso and chest when walking, achieving a "normal gait pattern:" a contra-lateral pattern of ambulation (when the right arm and left leg advance together followed by the left arm and right leg advancing together)?*

I always recommend that the patient become aware of her evolving pattern of movement throughout the day, and chart it down for herself. Similar to a diet log, she writes down her repeated patterns of motion using percentages to her best ability. It is hard to be aware of and attentive to your body while immersed in daily life. Knowing that she has a log to complete after the fact should stimulate her to be more in tune with her style of motion while interacting with the world.

> *Look around at the people you engage with often. Find someone who seems to be moving and interacting in a "balanced" way, using the three planes of movement equally. For example, moving her arms during interactions 33.3% front and back, 33.3% side-to-side, and 33.3% up and down. To get a better perspective on what "balanced" movement should look like, think of someone who is an "extreme" performer of the same motion (i.e. uses torso up and down 100% of the time in gestures or body posture) and compare this person's movement to your style. What did you learn from observing your movement style compared to others?*

Patient's response:
"I learned many things using my movement pattern log. I like sticking to my familiar movement pattern. It seems like I have my security

blanket surrounding my body when I am in my zone. I have a hard time being aware of the chest area and moving it from side-to-side. I feel more anxious when I need to start moving my rib cage area. It is difficult to modify my pattern. However, I am open to alterations since I feel that my chest is clogged and changing the way I handle and mobilize my body will be to my advantage."

Reader's response:

AWARENESS EXERCISE 8

> *The "outside-body" experience has to do with the way you feel in relation to where you are in space. For example, how much space do you occupy in different places: someone's house, your workplace, a classroom, etc.? How pronounced is your presence in the newly experienced space? The "inside-body" experience has to do with what you feel and sense happening within the body's physical limits. For example, I can expand my chest and feel warm and tender in my chest area, no matter where I am. The warmth and tenderness I experience heightens my awareness of the chest, thereby allowing me to be more fully present in whatever environment I am in.*

When a patient experiences "inside and outside body-experiences," she will often relate to what she feels and senses with regard to both the physical and emotional experiences of her body. In other words, she will feel her "physical experience" which has to do mostly with feeling the body physique (muscle tension, contraction, numbness, tingling, etc.), while the "emotional experience" relates mostly to the emotions she is aware of (fear, sadness, happiness, concern, etc.).

Patient's response:

"When I visit my parents' house, I feel my entire being present from the moment I step in the door. I am fully aware of my limbs and body, aware of being calm and loose. I feel a connection to the place which draws me in and I do not want to leave. In contrast, when I enter my work place that I dislike, I become dissociated from my body and am only conscious of the negative thoughts rushing through my head without being able to control them."

Reader's response:

AWARENESS EXERCISE 9

> *Are you able to evaluate your postures, gestures, and patterns of movement the way others evaluate you in terms of the usage of the vertical, sagittal and horizontal planes of motion? How objective are you in terms of knowing how you carry your body/self? To begin to answer these questions, you should first screen your body. Can you feel and sense all your body parts or not? For example, can you sense your feet, legs, belly area, chest, shoulders, arms, neck and face? What areas do you fail to notice?*

Patient's response:
"I can hardly sense my lower body from the pelvic area down. I am very aware of my chest, shoulders and arms. Those areas feel warm and heavy."

Reader's response:

In Summary

In order for the reader to utilize RiVision®, she must heighten her awareness of her posture, gestures, patterns of movement and quality of movement. Once the patient can identify her "baseline" or characteristic pattern of movement, then she can embark on altering it, if and when needed, when coping with daily life encounters. When practicing RiVision® and trying to heighten her bodily awareness, she should strive to recognize the difference between feeling and sensing her body in connection to her inside and outside "body-experiences" (*see* Awareness Exercise 8 above).

Grounding

As it applies to RiVision®, grounding (weight) refers to how much contact we experience with the ground. Is it strong and firm, or light and fine?

The variation in pressure (weight) adds to the range of what a person can do with her actual weight and muscular strength when resisting an object, situation or space. Lamb (1981) placed these on a continuum ranging from *firm*—strong resistance to weight and a movement sensation that feels heavy—to *fine*—light or weak resistance to weight and a movement sensation that is light. The purpose is to identify her typical movement pattern, and help her balance the usage of the motion within the continuum of firm to fine. This will enable her to expand and alter the pressure motion quality according to her needs. For example, when she approaches her baby daughter, she will use the more fine motion, and when she negotiates with her lawyer about serious legal matters, she can utilize the more firm motion.

"Grounding is connected to control," as one of my patients remarked. "When I am in control, my feet are stable on the ground; when I lose control, my feet are shaky on the ground."

It is important for the patient to feel her feet connected to the ground. Did she establish a partial connection to her base of support/ground or not? Did she feel that both her right and left foot were on the ground? Did she experience one foot more grounded than the other? How is the rest of the leg affected by the amount of grounding she experiences through the foot? Did she feel her feet in full contact with the ground and, if in partial contact, which part made the strongest contact with the ground? What is her physical impact on the ground: strong, light, no impact, just the right amount? When relating to the "Firm/Fine Scale" of motion, "firm" will be equal to zero and "fine" will be equal to ten. Check your grounding in everyday life encounters and rate it on this scale. The following are some exercises and the patient's responses given during the therapy sessions.

GROUNDING EXERCISE 1: GUIDED IMAGERY (SITTING OR STANDING POSITIONS)

> *Feel and sense each part of your foot and body. Can you feel or sense all parts of your body? Are there parts of your body or feet that you are not aware of? Now, see yourself entering different spaces: your home, your living room, a rented apartment, an elevator, an open meadow, a beach, a party place. What is your impact on the ground? Are you taking up a lot of space or a little? Are you impacting the ground you are stepping on? What is the impact of your presence on your surroundings? Are you pushing away with your presence? Are you attracting with your presence? Can you or would you like to change your impact on the earth/ground, at home or the office, or with your family?*

Patient's response:

"I do not want to make any impact when I go into a room with new people. I prefer to be almost invisible. I experience my impact on my surroundings in this new environment to be very minimal (possibly eight on the Firm/Fine Scale). This is a foreign place for me, which I translate to be a non-supportive one. Whereas, with my family, I feel that I take up more space and my steps are more grounded, as though each step makes a clear imprint on the floor."

Reader's response:

_____
_____
_____
_____
_____
_____
_____
_____
_____
_____

GROUNDING EXERCISE 2: GUIDED IMAGERY (STANDING POSITION)

> *Imagine your feet widening on top of the ground or extending into the ground. What do you feel and sense in your feet, legs, and your entire body when you imagine your feet widening on top of the ground or lengthening into the ground? Once you feel this, allow your feet to return to the normal physical limits of the body.*
>
> *Imagine that roots are growing from your heels. They develop into the ground as far as they can grow. Allow them to grow both to the sides and downward to the center of the earth. What do you feel and sense in your feet, legs, and your entire body? Once you have felt the sensation, have the roots return into your heels.*
>
> *Imagine your toes and the balls of your feet growing while the rest of the foot stays the same size. What do you feel and sense happening to your center of gravity (CG) and the rest of the body? Next try to imagine enlarging the heel area while the front and mid-part of the foot stays the same. What do you feel and sense happening to your CG and the rest of the body? Finally, return to the normal physical limits of the body.*

Patient's response:

"Both the imaginative roots exercise and the enlargement of my feet exercise grounded me. I was fully connected to the surface I was standing on. I felt stronger and more present."

Reader's response:

_____
_____
_____
_____
_____
_____

Cont'd...

Cont'd...

GROUNDING EXERCISE 3: PHYSICAL THERAPY

> *Stand with your feet apart. Feel and sense your body. Correct the space between your feet to make sure it is the most comfortable for you. Then, start shifting your weight from the right foot to the left. How did it feel while and after you were doing the movement? Compare the two sides of the body, sensing one segment at a time.*
>
> *Continue shifting your weight from side-to-side. Notice how far you can shift. Are you symmetrical? How does the shifting make you feel?*
>
> *Try lifting one leg at a time off the ground and then going back to full contact. Compare and relate to less or more stability in relation to your contact with the ground. What do you feel and sense? Notice what is happening to the rest of the body when you lose some contact with the ground.*
>
> *Walk around the room using big and then small steps. March stomping like a soldier and then softly like a cat. Walk with a three foot wide space between your feet (as if you have a beach ball between your legs) and then in a narrow stance with the feet touching each other.*

Patient's response:

"I was shaky when I needed to shift my weight from side-to-side. I was afraid of losing my balance and my sense of self. It reminded me of the way I feel when I am around my demanding father. I am not stable on my two feet. After practicing the shifting weight exercises for two months I felt more in control and I tried evaluating what was happening to me when I was around my father. I felt that I was more secure on my feet and the level of my anxiety decreased somewhat."

Reader's response:

In Summary

When using RiVision®, the reader needs to pay attention to how everyday life interactions with people or situations affect your patient's stability and balance. The therapy will propel her to evaluate, acknowledge and modify her pattern of movement to better serve her in relation to her surroundings. She will have a more "balanced" usage of fine and firm movements, and decreased bodily discomfort.

How grounded is she when sitting, standing and walking? Evaluate if she feels more or less secure, present and in control in different postures, gestures, and circumstances. Which movements make her feel more or less stable on the ground in everyday life situations? How can she modify her stance, emotionally and physically, in everyday life situations? For example, she can develop her awareness of what she experiences when placed in unfamiliar versus familiar environments. In an unfamiliar situation, with people she has never met before, she may feel foreign, tense and not connected to the ground. In a familiar situation, with beloved family or friends, she may feel significantly more secure and in full contact with the ground. These two different circumstances may affect how much physical and emotional connection she has on the ground.

Pacing

As it applies to RiVision®, pacing (time) refers to the process of changing your tempo of accelerating or decelerating the speed of motion.

Lamb (1981) placed these motions on a continuum ranging from *sudden*—quick speed of movement in a short span of time—to *sustained*—slow speed of a movement during a long span of time with a feeling of endlessness. The purpose is to identify one's typical movement pattern, and help her balance the usage of the motion within the continuum of sudden to sustained. This will enable her to expand and alter the pressure motion quality according to her needs. For example, using sudden movement qualities may save a fallen object from breaking. Using sustained movement qualities may help a person in severe pain maneuver her body carefully and attentively.

RiVision® pays attention to how fast or slow, or sudden or sustained she moves her body and extremities in general. Does she tend to move faster or slower in a particular situation? If she does, we pay attention to which situation prompts her to move faster or slower. Is she aware of the tempo of her torso and extremities? Do her torso and extremities move in synchrony or not? When the torso moves fast, do the arms move fast as well? Does she feel comfortable with her movement quality or does she prefer to change it? When relating to the "Sudden/Sustained Scale" of motion, "sustained" will be equal to zero and "sudden" will be equal to ten. The following are some exercises with patient responses given during the therapy sessions.

PACING EXERCISE 1: BODY AWARENESS AND PHYSICAL THERAPY

> *Check your pacing while walking and rate it on the Sudden/Sustained Scale. Are you accelerating or decelerating? What is your prominent feature, your pacing style? How often do you change your natural/prominent pace? Is it hard for you to move at a slow pace or at a fast pace?*
>
> *While walking, on which occasion do you find yourself accelerating or decelerating? Next relate to your gestures—what is your dominant pace when you gesture, interact, or argue?*
>
> *When comparing your movement and pacing style to others, are you faster or slower than others? Are you using extreme pacing motion on the Sudden/Sustained Scale or are you within the normal and balanced range? Are there particular body parts that you use to pace yourself more than others?*

Patient's response:

"My general pacing style is on the high end of the speedy-sudden style of motion. I can attest to the fact that my mom used to beg me to slow down when I moved around her house. I used to visit her, as a young man living independently in my flat, and she would scream at me, "Slow down before I throw you out!" I use my arms to gesture and express myself more than other body parts and they seem to be prominent in pacing me."

Reader's response:

_____
_____
_____
_____
_____

Cont'd...

Cont'd...

PACING EXERCISE 2: PHYSICAL THERAPY

> *Practice varied tempos of movement of your extremities and entire body. Move through the range of fast to slow motions. Can you modify your pace? How much control do you have? Do you feel that your pace may hinder your ability to communicate efficiently with others? Do you feel that your tempo obstructs you in any way?*

Patient's response:

"I estimate my movement style on the Sudden/Sustained Scale as eight out of ten. I feel that since I am a sudden, fast mover I probably impose tension on my surroundings. Elements of unpredictability and inner tension may emanate from my style. Trying to learn the implications of my sudden rushed tempo, I observed my coworker, Jim's, style of movement. He appears to have three out of ten on the Sudden/Sustained Scale. His style manifests itself in the way he speaks, walks and gestures. At work, he moves in a graded, slower pace. It may explain why people feel comfortable around him, gathering by his desk more often than mine and sometimes seeking his advice. He gives the feeling that he is not in a rush and his movements are more sequential and ordered."

Reader's response:

PACING EXERCISE 3: GUIDED IMAGERY

> *Imagine moving in an empty room and notice the way you pace yourself. Then imagine five more people come into the same room and notice if your tempo has changed. Imagine yourself talking with them and getting along very well. Observe your style. Now, change the scenario and imagine arguing with the people in the room. Observe the change in your movement pacing style.*

Patient's response:

"It was clear to me that when I imagine myself alone in the room I moved slower than when I had five people around me. Once I saw them around me, I was more sudden and quick when moving and reacting. In a way, I was at a higher attention level. I imagined my pace even faster when we argued."

Reader's response:

In Summary

When using RiVision®, you ask the reader to acquire the tools to evaluate her dominant style of motion. The therapy will propel her to evaluate, acknowledge and modify her pattern of movement to better serve her, with a more balanced usage of the sudden and sustained movements in relation to her surroundings. When does she move faster or slower? Does her movement pace change based on the environment? Is she comfortable with her movement style? Would she like to be more in control of it? For example, knowing what makes her start moving in an antsy manner causing rapid, suddenly accelerated motions (that might have been inappropriate for the situation) can help her relate to her pace of motion better. If she realizes that her movement pace may be out of the norm, and possibly cause her bodily discomfort and pain, it may encourage her to attempt to modify her repetitive pattern.

Orienting

As it applies to RiVision®, orienting (space) refers to the process of directing ourselves in space: specifically whether we move in a straight, direct manner or in a flexible, indirect manner.

According to Lamb, when we use the space around us we can move in a direct or indirect manner. *Direct* movement is a straight line that is narrow and focused. *Indirect* movement is a flexible, wave-like motion with a movement sensation of pliant extension in space (Lamb, 1981). One of the purposes of RiVision® is to identify the typical movement pattern of the individual, and to assist in balancing the usage of the motion within the continuum of direct to indirect. This will enable the person to expand and alter the orienting movement quality according to her needs. For example, she will use a direct movement quality when approaching her children and teaching them essential facts of life, while using an indirect movement quality when she is not clear about a subject.

A patient can have different preferences when she negotiates her movement in space. We pay attention to how direct or indirect her movements are. Is she aware of her movement preference: direct or indirect? Is she bothered by her preference of movement in daily life encounters? Does she live in peace with her movement pattern? When relating to the "Direct/Indirect Scale" of motion, "direct" will be equal to zero and "indirect" will be equal to ten. Check your space/orienting in everyday life encounters and rate it on this scale. The following are some exercises and patient's responses given during the therapy sessions.

ORIENTING EXERCISE 1: BODY AWARENESS

> *Notice how you approach someone standing to your side or in front of you. Are your movements sharp and direct or wavy and broad as you approach this person?*

Patient's response:

"I found that my motions are very direct and sharp; the motions are precise, quick and straight toward the person I am approaching. I found that people tend to step backward when I approach them, as if they are keeping a distance from me. I never before understood why."

Reader's response:

_____
_____
_____
_____
_____
_____
_____
_____
_____
_____
_____
_____
_____
_____
_____
_____

ORIENTING EXERCISE 2: PHYSICAL THERAPY

> *Move in indirect/angular wider motions. Vary the quality of your movement in all your body parts and then for the entire body. For example, move your arms in a wavy, angular, soft and slower pace while talking. See if you can maneuver your arms differently. How do you feel? Are you having a hard time changing your prominent style?*

Patient's response:

"I have a very hard time altering my style. It feels as though I have no control and no one will listen to me. It feels fake and artificial. How can I make the change so I will be able to expand my repertoire?"

Reader's response:

_____
_____
_____
_____
_____
_____
_____
_____
_____
_____
_____
_____
_____
_____
_____
_____
_____

ORIENTING EXERCISE 3: PHYSICAL THERAPY

> *Continue practicing the "other style" in a very graded manner. For instance, practice the indirect/angular motions only 10% of the time. Then gradually increase the repetition of the practice. At this first stage, introduce the motion only when you feel secure to do so. It may help you to experiment with the direct and indirect motions when you are with close family members. Observe how they react to your movement style change, if at all. This change may take a long time to establish. Do not expect a sudden change.*

Patient's response:

"I practiced at home when my mom was around. At first, she was oblivious to my changed style of motion. After about three months she noticed a change in me. She described the change as me being more at ease with myself. She probably was right to some extent. I felt that the constant practice of the indirect and softer motions affected the way I felt in general. It was a revelation for me. I loved the softer, indirect motions. It helped me feel less anxious."

Reader's response:

In Summary

When using RiVision®, the reader should be able to analyze her prominent movement style in terms of direct and indirect orientation in movement. How often and to what degree does she use each quality of the movement? In which situation does she tend to be more direct or indirect? Is there a correlation between her intention or agenda and the usage of her space? For example, when she is more intense, she may tend to move abruptly from one movement to the other using direct, short motions. She may now realize that her movement inflicts tension upon her close surroundings and therefore she may become determined to soften her movements.

Knowing how she is affecting her surroundings and how her state of being affects her movement style will be a stepping-stone in her therapy. It will propel her to evaluate, acknowledge and modify her pattern of movement to better serve herself (possibly with a more "balanced" usage of direct and indirect movements, decreased bodily discomfort) in relation to her surroundings (it is easier to communicate with a person who uses a more "balanced" movement pattern).

Muscle Tension

As it applies to RiVision®, muscle tension (flow) refers to the amount of free or bound flow of movement.

All movement produces muscular tension. A muscle works by contracting (tensing) and exerting a pull on the bony lever to which it is attached. The effort elements according to Lamb (1981) are *bound flow*, which consists of the readiness to stop normal flux or the sensation of pausing the movement, and *free flow,* which consists of released flux or the sensation of fluid movement.

Muscular tension varies between patients and can vary within a person during the day. The following observations should be made: Is the patient aware of her bound and free flow of movement? Is she aware of her preference of muscle tension in relation to her environment? Is she able to control the amount of tension in her muscles? Is she bothered by her free or bound flow movements during each daily life encounter? Does her particular muscle tension tendency serve her well? Does she live in peace with her current muscle tension?

In the course of therapy, the patient will be encouraged to evaluate and modify her bound/free flow of movement to achieve a more balanced usage of the flow movement scale. She will be able to use various degrees of muscle tensions on different occasions without being "stuck" in a narrow range on the bound to free continuum. Possibly, a greater range in the usage of the muscle tension (flow) scale will provide a greater variability in the way she communicates and handles others. When relating to the "Free/Bound Flow Scale" of motion, "free" flow will be equal to zero and "bound" flow will be equal to ten. Check your muscle tension in everyday life encounters and rate it on this scale. The following are some exercises with patient's responses given during the therapy sessions.

MUSCLE TENSION EXERCISE 1: GUIDED IMAGERY (SITTING OR STANDING)

> *Imagine "oiling" your joints and muscles from the inside of your body to lubricate them. Now feel and sense your body. How does it feel? Is there any difference from before the "lubrication?" If there is no change, try to imagine "lubricating" from outside the body using ointments or lotions. Check again, how does it feel now?*
>
> *Imagine yourself standing in the middle of a meadow, moving like a blade of grass in the light breeze, using soft, fluid motions. Can you imagine the quality of your movements as a graceful blade of grass? If not, try to imagine moving like any other natural, soft form you can relate to. For example, I can imagine my arms moving like a dove's wings.*
>
> *Imagine a movement without actually moving your body. Can you imagine moving your arms up and down like real bird wings and feeling and sensing the quality of the motion, the air surrounding the motions, the temperature around your wings and yourself, and the sound of the flickering wings?*
>
> *Check what you feel and sense in your shoulders, neck, chest and arms. Check how much, if at all, you can get into the bird-like motion image in terms of the width and length of the movement.*

Patient's response:

"Oiling my joints" was an amazing feeling. I could sense how my joints were gradually becoming softer. Then, the image I had while in the meadow was of being a big condor gliding powerfully above my house. My wings were swinging up and down smoothly. I felt free and strong. I rarely feel like this. It was surprising to experience it. I wanted to hold onto the sensation forever.

Reader's response:

MUSCLE TENSION EXERCISE 2: BODY AWARENESS AND PHYSICAL THERAPY

Free flow motion encompasses softness and flexibility while the bound flow is more rigid and firm. Practice free flow (soft) versus bound flow (rigid) movement patterns. How would you define your "body state" on the Free/Bound Flow Scale?

Now, practice movements that begin free and become increasingly bound. Then move in the opposite direction, from bound movements to free.

Think of a person you know who demonstrates either extreme of rigidity or softness in movement.

How do you perceive yourself on the Free/Bound Flow Scale: at work, in tense situations, and at home?

Patient's response:
"I am more rigid in general, possibly seven on the Free/Bound Flow Scale. I believe my father is the rigid type. I sense his rigidity in his gestures and facial expressions. The rigidity I perceive from him makes my chest tighter and I have some difficulties freeing my torso when I am in his proximity. When I separate from him and I am with my girlfriend I feel freer in the chest area, able to breathe and move the ribcage with ease."

Reader's response:

___

Cont'd...

Cont'd...

MUSCLE TENSION EXERCISE 3: BODY AWARENESS AND PHYSICAL THERAPY

> Let us consider which body part is most involved in your movement, then evaluate the quality of that dominant body part's movement. For example, if you mostly move your arms, check whether the quality is more of the free or bound flow. Now, see if you have the capability to modify the quality of your arm movements. Evaluate again what happens to your free and bound flow when you are in particular situations. Pay closer attention to the quality of your motion in relationship to the circumstances.
>
> Now, find your specific cause-effect formula. For example, cause could be, "My boss repeats himself until I cannot tolerate his comments any more." The effect could be, "Tension builds in the base of my skull on the right side." Come up with several cause-effect relationships from daily life situations.

Patient's response:

"In general, my neck gets the most tension. The pain accompanying the tension starts at the bottom of the neck and crawls up to the base of my skull. I realize that when I encounter my dad, the tension builds up rapidly in the neck and chest areas. When I am not with him and I am with my girlfriend, the tension subsides significantly. Another cause-effect example is from my work. When I am with my boss I start experiencing the tension building up rapidly, but when I am talking with my coworker, Emily, who is a soft-spoken, sweet human being, my body softens and I do not experience discomfort in the neck or chest area."

Reader's response:

_____
_____
_____
_____

Cont'd...

In Summary

In RiVision®, the reader needs to pay attention to the quality of her motions. How free or bound are her motions? Being fully aware of her pattern of movement in relation to her experiences can be the key for altering her movement style if it is hindering well-being and daily function. Finding the cause-effect relationship between restrictive and negative body manifestations (like pain and tension) and personal interactions in different environments (calm versus tense environments) may be crucial in breaking the vicious cycle of negative experiences. For example, she will be able to notice that she tends to move in a bound quality of motion when she is around a threatening parent's figure and she has the capacity of changing her movement flow under the right circumstances.

In this chapter, I have outlined the five motion factors (awareness, grounding, pacing, orienting and muscle tension), including patient responses. The reader was encouraged to fill in her response when it is relevant to her. In the following chapter, four representative case studies will describe, in a step-by-step fashion, the development of the treatment protocols.

Chapter 5

Case Studies: Treatment Goals, Exercises and Outcomes

CASE STUDY # 1—BETTY

As we grow in age and experience, our body and mind register the information most pertinent to us on different levels, whether subconscious or conscious. But we often lose the sense of all the knowledge already stored in our body level. We block that knowledge, not wanting to re-experience traumas, fears and even excitement that our vulnerable selves have gone through. The question is how to better grasp and assimilate our difficult experiences so that we can overcome the blockages they create in our lives.

I met Betty, 23 years old, when she was referred to me with a diagnosis of shoulder and neck pain for the prior six months. When she entered the room I saw a smiling young woman with a pleasant demeanor, of average height, who had long hair and was chubby (Figs. 5.1 and 5.2). She was pursuing a Bachelor's degree in Art, played the guitar and performed as a part time singer.

When I asked about her family, she described her parents who still lived together but had been emotionally separated from each other for many years. Her father frequently belittled her mother and he attempted suicide once. Her 60-year-old mother had chronic leukemia, was on and off chemotherapy, depressed and overweight. Her mother needed attention but did not have many real friends. Betty stated that she tried giving her mother as much attention as she could.

"My father was mean to my mother," Betty explained. He denied that she had cancer and did not attend to her mother's needs, while respecting Betty for being independent and moving forward. Betty pursued a Bachelor's degree in Art. She worked hard and supported

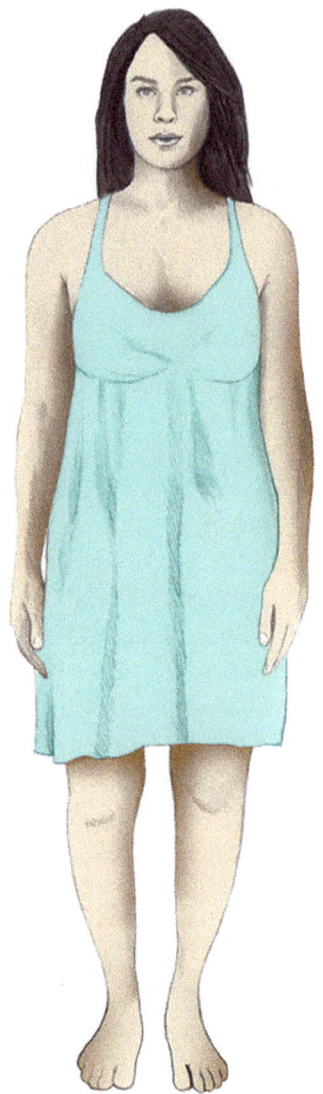

Fig. 5.1: Betty's front view.

herself without their help. Betty's sister distanced herself from the entire situation, was married, and seemed to Betty to be non-emotional and reluctant to deal with their father's issues.

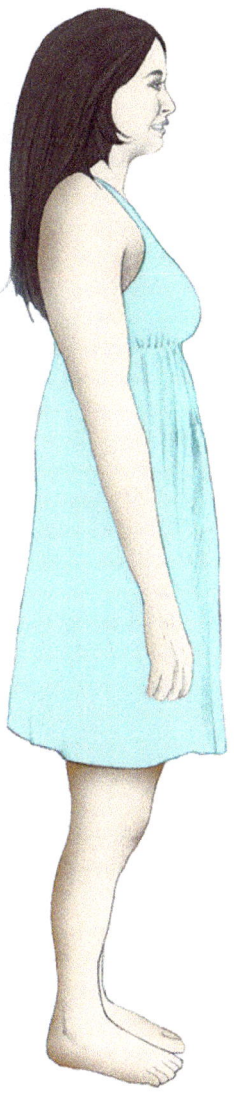

Fig. 5.2: Betty's side view.

Betty told me that since childhood she had been dissociated from her body. According to Betty, her father would scream and yell at her until she cried. Eventually she learned to disconnect her body from

64   *Moving Pain Away-RiVision®: An Innovative Physical Therapy Method*

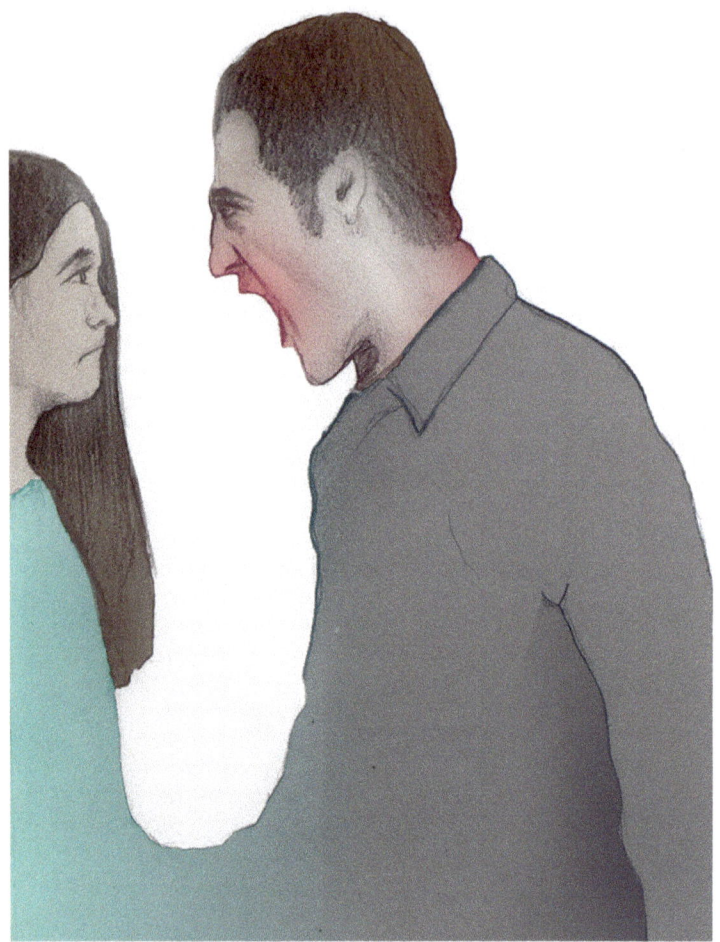

Fig. 5.3: Father screams at Betty.

her feelings and let him yell (Fig. 5.3). She added that she could not and would not cry anymore. When she was training to be an opera singer, she would dissociate from her body while singing on stage (Fig. 5.4). She explained that she would be standing on stage and performing, but would not feel herself singing. "I wouldn't be there at all. Actually I would be standing outside of myself and watching my body on stage."

Case Studies: Treatment Goals, Exercises and Outcomes **65**

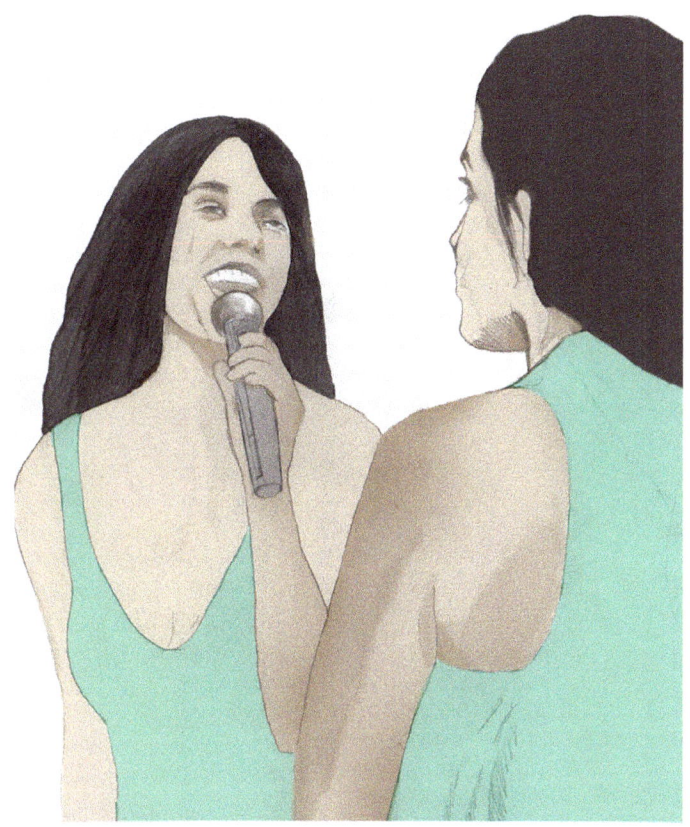

Fig. 5.4: Betty dissociates from her body while singing.

Betty told me that two years ago her father had a heart attack and double bypass surgery. This was a major wake-up call for her because she was finally informed of the long family history of heart disease, prompting her to think about losing weight. At that time, she added, she was full of anger and fear surrounding her relationship with her father, as well as her many failed relationships with men.

In the initial stage of therapy, Betty and I had two main goals in mind: to help her with the shoulder pain and to increase her ability to feel and sense her body. Once the shoulder got better in terms of increased range of motion and decreased pain, I shifted my goal and concentrated more on the entire person. My idea was to help Betty increase her awareness of her experiences of bodily tension, frustration, fear and resentment, so she could tap into what she feels and senses in the moment. We began with physical therapy and guided imagery. Betty was open to going through these therapies, which enabled her to feel and sense further what happens to herself. Without her openness and belief in the possibilities these processes held for her, we would not have found change and success.

GUIDE TO BETTY'S TREATMENT

Encounter I

Betty said she was willing to do all that it would take to heal. She was open to criticism and enthusiastic about seeing changes. However, her body was flooded with anger and frustration toward her parents. She expressed various negative emotions repetitively.

Goal

Enhance her body awareness to various emotions and sensations (e.g. frustration, fear, tension, softness, etc.)

Body Awareness Exercises

Exercise 1

> Therapist (T): *"Try to notice the sensations of your body: starting from your feet and working your way up, how do the different parts of your body feel physically (e.g. tension, spaciousness, tingling, contraction, etc.)?"*

Betty: "My chest is like a ball and there is a large, black stain in the chest going up to my throat (Fig. 5.5)."

Guided Imagery

Exercise 1

> T: *"Now, try to imagine yourself in the presence of your father and become aware of your body's physical sensations and emotions in this imaginary situation."*

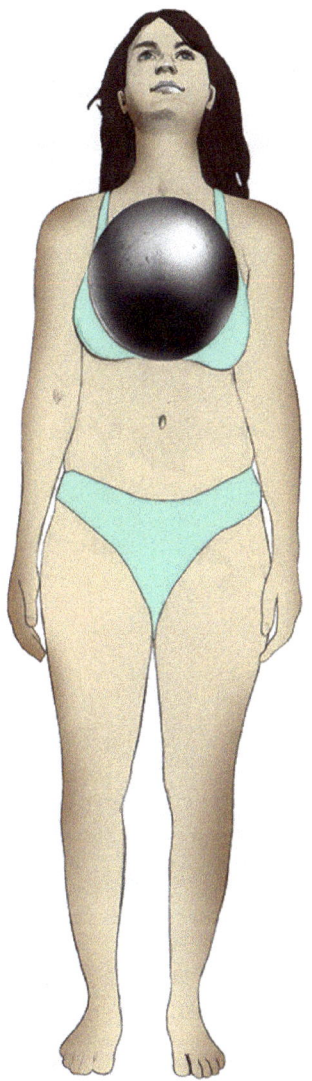

Fig. 5.5: Betty imagines a large ball inside her chest.

Betty: "I am trying to talk with him, but he does not listen, like always. I am frustrated and tense. I feel it in the upper body: chest, throat and neck."

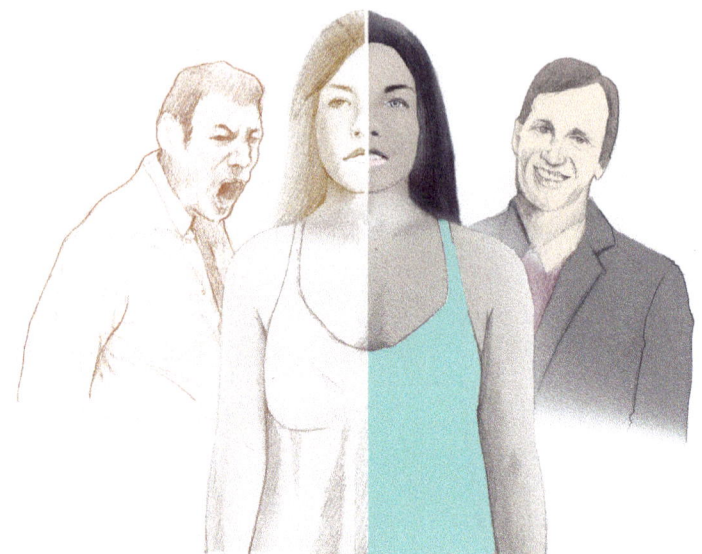

Fig. 5.6: Betty's biological father and "preferred" father.

Exercise 2

> T: *"Try to remove your father from your imaginary field and bring in a different person, a 'preferred' father image (Fig. 5.6)."*

After a few minutes Betty responded: "I feel much better, less tense, my upper body is looser."

Exercise 3

The next step was a complex activity since T was asking Betty to bring together two different images and relate to both at the same time. This could interfere with the clarity of the image in some people so T suggests using it only with those patients who are more open to or practice guided imagery (Betty, for example, being a musician, came in with a strong sense of her imaginative powers).

> T: *"Try to imagine both of these father Figures around you, and try to notice your sensations and emotions as you relate to each one of them separately (Fig. 5.6)."*

Betty: "I see my father on my right; the right side of my face is heavy. The 'preferred' father is on my left and the left side of my face feels more relaxed."

Exercise 4

> T: *"Staying in this imaginary shared space, can you talk with both men? Can you conduct a conversation with them?"*

After a short pause Betty said: "I am having a very hard time doing this."

> T: *"Okay. Let's leave it for the time being."*

Encounter II

Betty told T that her father had asked her to come with him to lunch while she was visiting her mom. She described not wanting to leave her mom alone, but nevertheless took up his offer and went with him. She succumbed to him while knowing that her mom needed her and wanted her around.

Goal

Heighten awareness of her emotions and sensations when she does something that is not right for her.

Guided Imagery

Exercise 1

> T: *"See yourself situated between your mother and father (Fig. 5.7): check how your spine looks to you. Is it straight? Tilted to one side? Strong or weak? Stable or not? Can you sense the temperature of your body and spine? How does the rest of your body feel?"*

Betty described that her spine was awkward and weak. The temperature inside her body was warm and her body did not feel intact. "For example, I feel only a slight connection between my muscles and tendons to the spine."

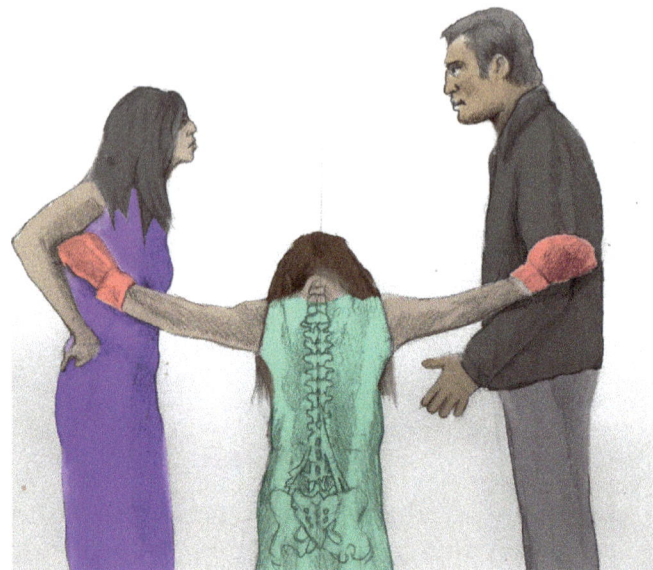

Fig. 5.7: Young Betty in between her parents.

> T: *"Now imagine yourself turning 30 years old, behaving in a more mature manner and responding accordingly (Fig. 5.8). How would you have reacted or responded if you had been fully mature and rational? Check back to your body using guided imagery. Notice your emotions (feel) and sensations (sense)."*

Betty reported that her body grew and expanded in a good way. "I felt stable, firm with a strong spine. I could imagine being able to listen to what I needed to do and not what he wanted me to do."

Encounter III

Betty presented her concern that it was difficult for her to make decisions and choose between right and wrong. We all struggle with decisions and try to choose wisely between various options. Decision-making is a process which can shake us up significantly; bring about fear, indecisiveness, anxiety, worries and negative feelings.

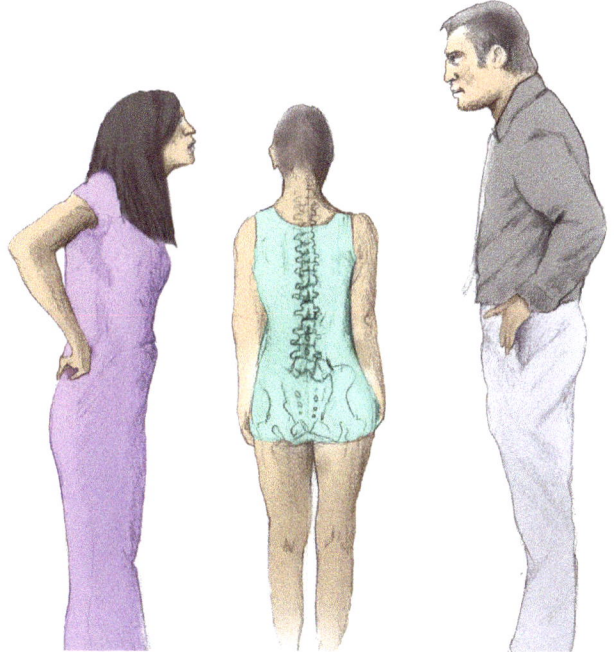

Fig. 5.8: More mature Betty in between her parents.

Goal

Heighten awareness of her bodily experience when she is clear or unclear about making a decision.

Guided Imagery

Exercise 1

> T: *"Imagine a situation where you are struggling between siding with one person or another (do not relate to your parents). Imagine dividing your acquaintances into two smaller groups: one group represents those you do not want to be associated with, while the other group represents people with whom you want proximity (Fig. 5.9). Now, imagine yourself interacting with either group. What is happening in your body? What do you feel (emotions) and sense (physical sensations)?"*

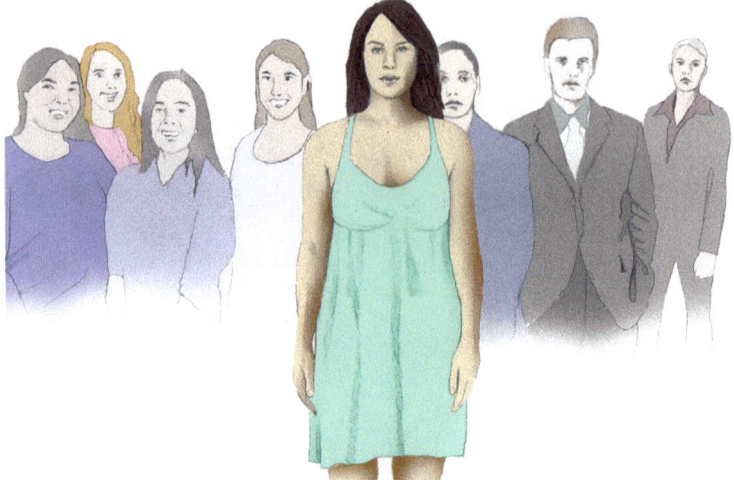

Fig. 5.9: Betty's acquaintances—two opposite groups.

Betty: "When I sided with my favorite group of people my body was calmer and more expanded in the chest area. When I was with the ones whom I disagree with, my body was tighter, tenser, my chest was narrower and it was harder for me to breathe (Figs. 5.10A and B)."

> T: *"So now you were able to make a clear distinction between how you are experiencing your body with the two opposite types of groups. Being able to notice what happens to your body in relation to social interaction made a different impact upon you. See if you encounter similar experiences more often during the day."*

Encounter IV

Betty's mom had poor posture: she was bent forward with curved-in shoulders that allowed minimal torso, shoulder and neck mobility. Betty suffered from shoulder pain due to strain in both shoulders. At the first stage of physical therapy we used conventional methods to try to alleviate her shoulder pain. For example, we used therapeutic exercises, soft tissue and joint mobilizations, and ultrasound to help with the shoulder tendinitis in the front part of the shoulders.

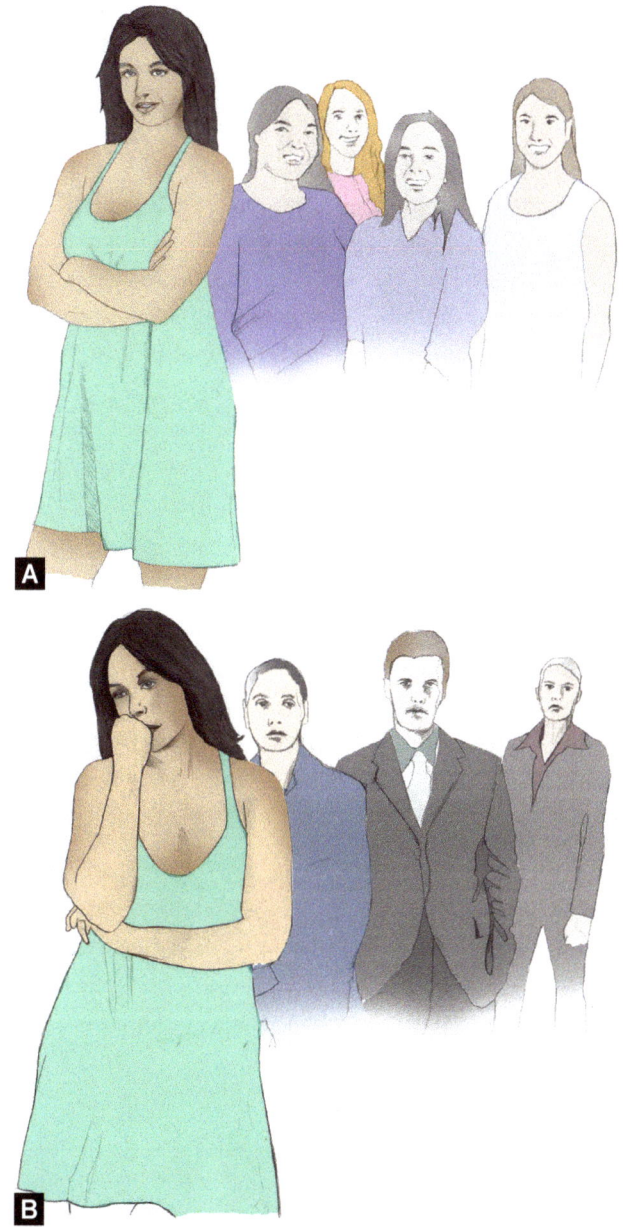

Figs. 5.10A and B: (A) Betty's experience "with my favorite group", (B) Betty's experience "with ones I disagree with".

As Betty's range of motion increased as well as her flexibility and general awareness of how to sit properly, we realized that there was more to the "physical treatment" that was keeping her body down. She was consciously able to erect her spine using the exercises and body awareness techniques we utilized; however, it was an artificial act on her part. The spine straightening and the expansion of the chest were executed upon her will and determination despite something inside her that kept her down. She knew that she needed to help her upper body pain by erecting her spine and maintaining particular positions of her scapula, chest, shoulders and torso, but she did it because it was taught by T. Something deep inside her was keeping her down and we set out to find what it was.

Goal

Changing posture, grounding body and erecting upper body.

Guided Imagery

Exercise 1

> T: *"Imagine developing roots from the heels of your feet (Fig. 5.11). How far do they grow? Do they grow equally on both sides, or not? Move to one side (right) then the other (left)."*

Betty described that her body felt grounded (connected to the floor/base of support) and her upper body was very tense. In a way her body was divided into two parts: her lower body, from her hips down to her toes, was firmly placed on the ground while the upper body, from the belly up to her head, was tense, condensed and frozen.

Exercise 2

> Since the upper body needed to "unfreeze" in order for her to feel better, T asked Betty to imagine expanding her shoulders by broadening to both sides, creating circular motions back and forth with her shoulders and expanding her chest and arms.

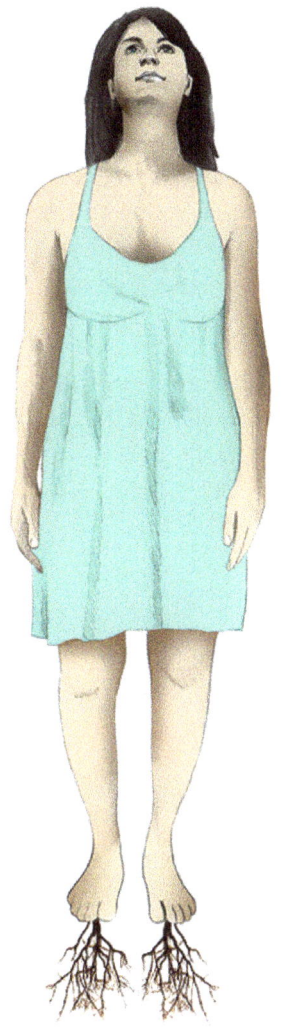

Fig. 5.11: Betty's imaginative roots.

Betty responded by saying that her spine felt very curved. She felt the tension in her spine more so after doing the upper body guided imagery motions.

> T asked why Betty was in this curved position?

Betty explained that despite the fact that she does not know what prompts her exaggerated curvy spine she noticed her tensed spine and body.

> T: *"Who in your family has a similar posture?"*

Betty said that as far as she could analyze postures, her mom's posture is very much like hers. "The difference between us is in the amount of flexibility. I am more flexible."

> T: *"Could you evaluate the differences between your postures (Fig. 5.12)? What are the respective postures (mom's and hers) trying to convey? Is there a statement made by the posture? Can you find your own style based on your posture? Can you find your mom's style based on her posture?"*

Betty responded by saying that she was not sure how she could find her own style.

Goal

Find her body style.

Guided Imagery and Physical Exercises

Exercise 1

> In order to facilitate Betty's body awareness and ability to identify her own style of movement/posture, T asked her to imagine her spine moving like a wave. The wave motion was initiated at the tailbone moving up to the base of the skull, forming an elongation in the spine.

Betty was excited to inform me that her spine was loose and free and the guided imagery facilitated the freedom of the entire body.

> T instructed her in utilizing the "wave-like" movement (imagine it) when she sensed her tension building up, i.e. with coworkers and friends.

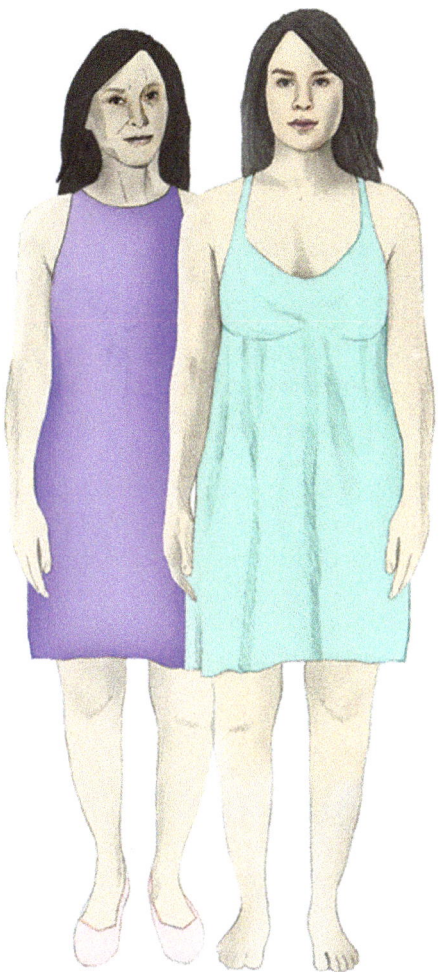

Fig. 5.12: Betty and her mom's similar postures.

Exercise 2

T encouraged her to check what her posture was trying to convey to her and to others, and whether she liked this posture or not. Would she rather modify it or not? If she could alter her posture when she was determined to do so, was she capable? T further asked her to check how her posture changes in different environments.

Encounter V

Betty was overwhelmed at times by the depth of inquiry entailed in this work. However, she was fully cooperative and easily took in feedback from T. During the first several meetings she was moderately anxious and concerned about how good she would be. T encouraged her to concentrate simply on the actions without worrying about the end results. My repeated reassurance played an important role in supporting her.

Betty described how this holistic approach combining dance/movement therapy (DMT) and guided imagery forced her to be more in tune with whom she wanted to be and whom she would like to have as her friends. The therapy assisted her in being more selective and assertive about her choices. However, Betty still struggled with various emotions, such as emptiness, anger, a need for fulfillment, pain, no satisfaction, confusion and painful feelings about her boyfriend. She explained searching for direction in life professionally and personally.

Betty expressed that she did not know how to evaluate herself as a human being. She felt that she was not familiar with herself enough, not clear about how she handled relationships, her flaws and strengths, work relations and being independent.

Goal

Develop her personal identity.

Dance/Movement Therapy

Exercise 1

> *Betty was confused regarding a wide variety of issues related to her growth and well-being. T instructed her to dance in her own style, to form a movement that was hers, to form a gesture that was hers, to form a facial expression that represented her and to identify a posture that was hers. T continued to facilitate her identification with her style and distinguish between it and the styles of others. "Dance like your mom/dad/sibling/favorite friend/non-favorite friend/perfect you/ugly you/ trouble maker you/good you/optimal you." T gave the following instructions:*

Cont'd...

Cont'd...

> 1. Dance who you are right now (Fig. 5.13A).
> 2. Dance who you would like to be in the near future (Fig. 5.13B).
> 3. Dance who you would be in 2, 5, 10, 20 years from now (Fig. 5.13C).
> 4. Dance alone on this earth and notice what you feel and sense.
> 5. Dance with good friends and pay attention to what you notice about your body.

Guided Imagery

Exercise 1

T asked Betty the following questions.

> *In sitting position:*
> *Where in your body is your "inner wisdom area"?*
> *Where in your body is your "inner knowledge area"?*
> *Where in your body is your area of clarity?*
> *Where in your body is your center of being?*
> *Where in your body are your centers of weakness, strength, anger, sadness, frustration, fear, joy, optimism and beauty?*

Exercise 2

> *While walking:*
> T: "See yourself as 'perfect you' walking alone in the desert while your boyfriend walks toward you and then away. Next, picture your 'ideal man' walking toward you and then away."

Betty described that when her boyfriend came toward her she grew and when he left she collapsed. When the "ideal man" approached her she not only felt herself growing taller but also expanding with confidence to the sides of her body and looking better than when she was imagining her encounter with her boyfriend.

Exercise 3

> T: *"Imagine you are a tree—what kind? How many roots, branches?"*

Betty described a soft and extremely small Bonsai tree with no flowers, a narrow trunk, and small, narrow branches.

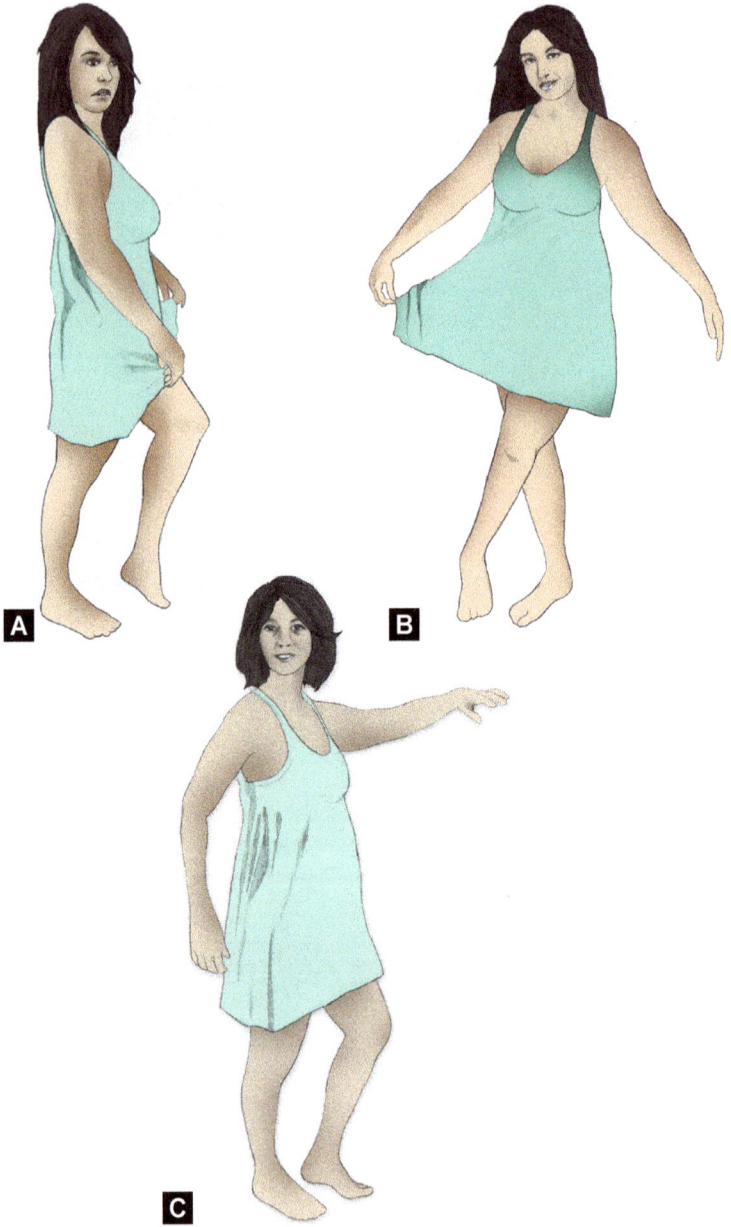

Figs. 5.13A to C: (A) Betty dancing now, (B) Betty imagines herself dancing in the near future, (C) Betty imagines herself dancing in the far future.

T: *"How would you like to see your tree in one year from now?"*

Betty: "I want to be more beautiful and noticed like a moderate-sized Redbud tree covered with purple flowers in early spring."

T: *"Find yourself in the middle of an orchard. See your fruits and flowers. Then collect your fruits and organize yourself as a new, strong and stable version of your original tree. Feel it."*

Betty: "I see myself developing into a larger and wider Redbud tree standing in the center of the orchard and feeling entitled to be in the center."

T: *"Imagine seeing yourself/body in the orchard growing roots from the heels of your feet. Then find your 'center of being.' Let your center move back and forth without losing your ground."*

Betty responded that she now felt more connected to the ground so that it was hard to shift her out of balance. She felt that she was being placed more securely and firmly on this earth, and that her stance was becoming harder to influence.

Encounter VI

Betty stated that she felt that her present friends were not suited for her. Previously she believed that she could not judge their characters objectively and was biased due to her vulnerability and neediness. Now she felt that she was able to judge, evaluate, and choose more appropriately than before. T encouraged Betty to ponder about: "What is a good friend? How many do you need? Why do you need a particular friend? If you define development as greater self-esteem, beauty, confidence and strength, have you been improving in this process so far?" Betty felt that she still needed to develop tools that would help her choose the right friends.

Goal

To enhance self-esteem, confidence and self-worth.

Guided Imagery

Exercise 1

> T: *"Imagine yourself in a new place (job or social setting). What color is emanating from your body?"*

Exercise 2

> T: *"Notice your emotions and bodily sensations."*

Exercise 3

> T: *"Where do you feel and sense the strength, inner power, knowledge (wisdom), experience or lack of experience, weakness, fear, anxiety, hope and patience located in your body?"*

Exercise 4

> T: *"Imagine the person whom you perceive as respecting you the most gazing at you and the person respecting you the least gazing at you. What happens to your body?"*

Betty described that she felt the most expanded when her mom and people who respected her looked at her. "My chest is wider and less tense."

Exercise 5

> T: *"Practice the 'Regal Pose.' Notice your emotions and physical sensations as if you were a queen wearing the appropriate attire, using queenly manners and feeling like royalty (Fig. 5.14). Repeat doing so throughout the entire day."*

Betty stated that one of the most important things she had learned from RiVision® was that she was a princess learning to become a queen. That meant that she could be proud to be in her body: she could sit, walk, run and do everything with perfect posture and a sense of dignity. She felt and sensed herself as being beautiful and worthy of attention, love and affection. It did not matter to her that she was somewhat overweight. She genuinely was able to love and respect herself.

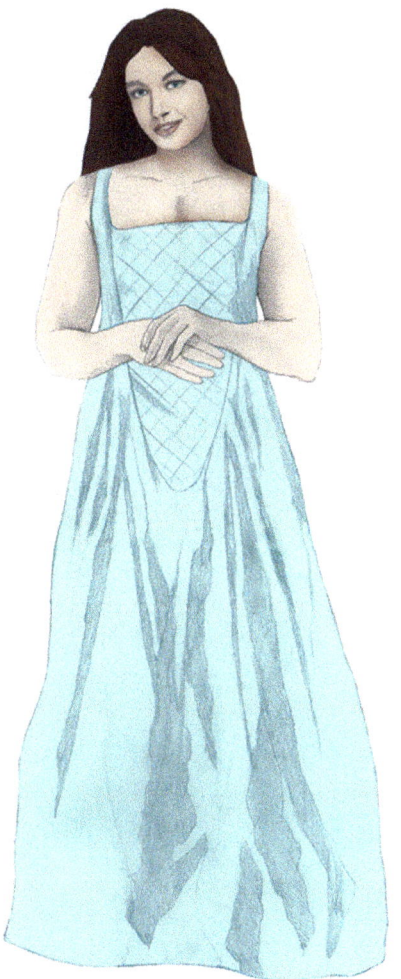

Fig. 5.14: Betty's "Regal Pose."

Dance/Movement Therapy

Exercise 1

T asked Betty to focus her attention on the elements that hindered her from feeling good about herself. T directed Betty to experience and explore via DMT which emotions limited her motion.

During a DMT session, Betty recognized emotional weakness in her upper body and arms, and a corresponding inability to execute a strong motion with her arms.

> *Then T introduced role-play to the dance therapy session to stimulate a changing experience that would later lead to feeling stronger in the upper body.*

Initially, the challenge for Betty was to feel and connect to the area that "the weakness" occupied within her body. Then Betty began to train herself, with the assistance of imagery and music, to support, build up and modify her upper body self-perception. She was encouraged to move with gestures and motions that would elicit more power and strength in her upper body.

During later stages, we explored a large array of feelings and emotions during the movement sessions to discern where each one was located in Betty's body and how each one influenced her general state of mind, movement patterns and posture.

> *In the final stage of this sequence T asked Betty to try to feel and sense being and moving like a queen, reinforcing a change in the way she perceived herself in relation to her body.*

Encounter VII

Betty had a tendency to shift moods relatively quickly. For example, she would suddenly burst into laughter after being still and quiet for a while.

Goal

Stabilize mood/reaction to fewer ups and downs.

Dance/Movement Therapy

Exercise 1

> *Experience extremes—T asked Betty to dance the following opposite states: loose/tight, fast/slow, direct/indirect, straight forward/roundabout, quiet/noisy, soft/rigid, focused/blurry, all over body motion/separate individual motions.*

Exercise 2

> *Experience gradual shifts in position*—T asked Betty to check which movements/gestures she uses in everyday life when walking, talking, interacting with people, laughing, reflecting, etc. T asked how often she executed a movement/mood with extreme intensity. Which part(s) of her gesture and motions require moderation? Which motions require modifications? Could she moderate her movements by herself?

Betty stated that she was not aware of the fact that she had sudden and extreme mood shifts. Practicing the opposite states (exercise #1) and the gradual shifts (exercise #2) heightened her self-awareness. She was surprised, slightly amused and disappointed by the way she found herself to be after so many years; she realized how awkward and different her actions and reactions were in comparison to other people's; and, most dramatically, how much more work was ahead of her. With her will to change for the better and T's support and encouragement, Betty was leaping forward and progressing nicely after five months of treatment. Her sudden mood shifts and bursts of movements diminished. She developed more control, graded intensity and greater balance of her movement pattern. She felt more charming, beautiful, worthy of love, and appreciative of herself.

Her treatment lasted several months since we simultaneously employed various modalities that required an extensive period of time to effect a positive change. In the DMT part of the treatment, intervention involved much assessment of movement style limitations, insight and change. One also has to positively accept that the process of altering an embedded part of oneself is gradual and slow.

CASE STUDY # 2—WEN

Wen had been suffering from asthma for many years. She originally came to treatment because she broke her foot. Once her foot got better I offered to work on her asthma condition (Fig. 5.15). I was struck by her posture and the shape of her chest because she seemed not to be breathing, and even if she attempted to expand her rib

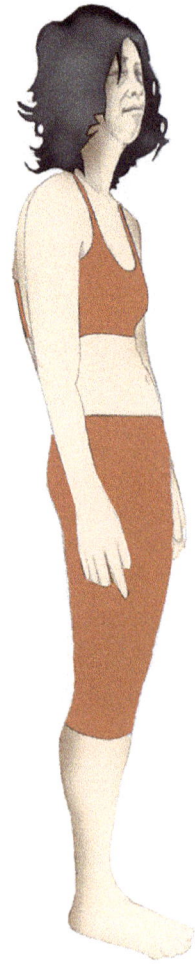

Fig. 5.15: Wen's posture before treatment.

cage, there was very limited motion. Tension in muscles can be distributed throughout the body in different locations. Stress and anxiety can cause physiological changes that may provoke asthma attacks, increased muscle spasm and pain in the chest area. Initially, I did not evaluate her chest/rib motion as a physical therapist might have done. I relied on my general impression that her chest seemed frozen and trusted my response, which was based on what I saw and experienced in my own body. I felt in her a sense of being stuck, sucked downward, feeling very heavy, dry and congested.

At the time I did not know whether Wen's chest area would respond positively to a new approach that I had developed for treating asthmatics, but had yet to try out. The combined method using DMT, guided imagery and hands-on techniques allowed me to experience her totality and not necessarily focus on the asthma, while promoting faster healing. It was also beneficial that Wen was very cooperative and eager to try the new approach.

Wen described that she had been using her inhaler on a regular basis for many years. She used it on average three times a day. Her asthma worsened in cold weather and only warm weather helped somewhat. Objective evaluation revealed a curved forward chest and kyphotic upper body. Upon palpation of her chest area, I found moderate muscle spasm around the entire chest and rib cage musculature.

Initially, Wen was quick to use the method, apply several techniques and was very attentive to our work. The first stage of the treatment included therapy: joint and soft tissue mobilization in the rib cage area, sternum bone, and cervical and thoracic spine. Touch and palpation of the vulnerable area was very significant. Wen said that she felt she could expand her lungs and chest a bit more after each treatment, and more air was being exchanged in each breath.

My current goals were to enhance awareness and facilitate change in Wen's posture and breathing habits. I also wanted to increase her awareness and understanding of the connection between breathing patterns, posture, movement patterns and traumatic life experiences. From the beginning of the treatment, I noticed a gradual slow change and, after about two months, she needed to use her inhaler

50% less often than before. Incorporating work with DMT and guided imagery convinced her that a physical change could take place and her ribs and lungs could work more efficiently. It boosted her confidence and gave us some fuel to move forward.

GUIDE TO WEN'S TREATMENT

Encounter I

Wen experienced and imagined her chest as small, pushed in, "frozen" with lack of mobility. She described that she had this experience for as long as she could recall.

Goal

Alter her chest image.

Guided Imagery

Exercise 1

> *Therapist (T) asked Wen to envision her chest area from the inside and from the outside. For example, T asked, "What picture do you get of your right and left lungs if you observe them with an imaginative magnifying glass from the inside of the chest? What picture do you get if you observe the lungs with an imaginative magnifying glass from outside the chest?"*

In order to accomplish the goal of altering her chest image, she needed to be able to perceive the tight chest as being looser from different angles. The sternum and the front of the chest were the first target.

Exercise 2

> *T guided Wen who was lying supine to imagine her chest expanding up to the ceiling of the room and then returning to the normal physical limits of the chest (Fig. 5.16). She needed to report how she felt and sensed the area after practicing the exercises several times.*

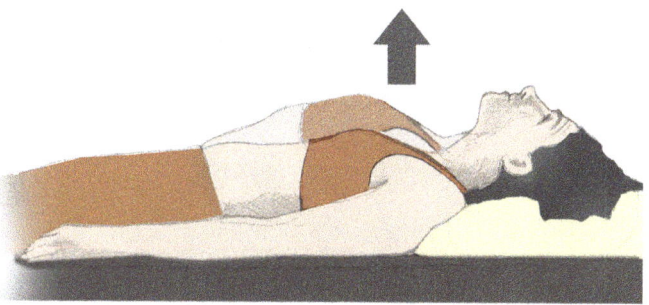

Fig. 5.16: Wen imagines expanding her chest upward.

Exercise 3

> *Next, T guided Wen to experience the expansion on both sides of the chest (Fig. 5.17), then from the back down toward the floor. Each motion was first performed separately, then we tried to combine directions and see whether it brought less or more relaxation to the area.*

In general, Wen said that her chest got light in color, larger, freer and looser. In a later point in the treatment, we utilized two additional exercises based on the book "Asthma-free in 21 days" by Kathryn Shafer and Fran Greenfield (2000): The Golden Inhaler (p. 57) and The Golden Bellows (p. 59).

Exercise 4

> *The Golden Inhaler—*
> *"Intention: To give you a way to reduce or replace the use of your regular inhaler.*
> *Frequency: Use this exercise as needed or whenever you reach for your regular inhaler. It gives you a choice and helps you to become your own authority.*
> *Note: There is no introductory breathing process for this exercise.*
> *Whenever you need to use the inhaler, reach for it, hold it in your hand, and then stop for an instant. In that instant of stopping (and before you do anything with the inhaler), close your eyes and imagine that you are bringing a golden inhaler into your mouth,*

Cont'd...

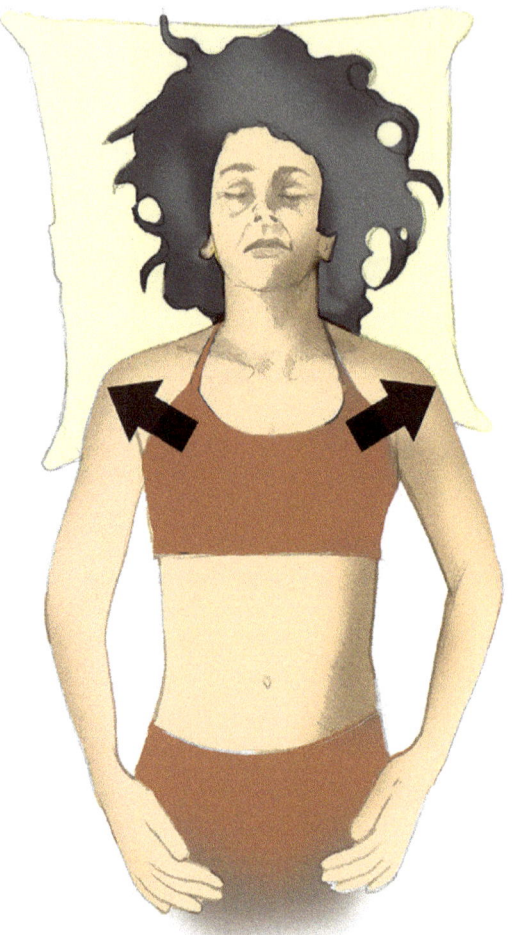

Fig. 5.17: Wen imagines expanding her chest sideways.

Cont'd...

> or however you use it. Take the number of puffs that you ordinarily use, and see this coming out as a blue spray, which you ingest. See it filling your lungs and bronchi with blue light, allowing you to breathe normally. Then open your eyes and complete the action in any way you see it."

Exercise 5

> *The Golden Bellows—*
> "*Intention:* To strengthen and heal the respiratory system. To increase lung capacity.
> *Frequency:* If you are experiencing respiratory discomfort, use once every hour or two while awake, up to two minutes at a time. If breathing is normal, use once in the morning and once at night.
> Close your eyes and breathe out three times. Imagine your lungs as a pair of golden bellows. As you breathe in, see, sense, and feel the bellows filling with white light and expanding. See and feel your chest expanding at the same time.
> As you exhale, see the bellows contracting forcibly, pushing out the impure air through your mouth. See this air being emitted as gray smoke and drifting away into the atmosphere. At the same time, see and sense your chest contracting. Now repeat this process up to five more times before opening your eyes. As you do this, know that your lungs are working rhythmically, filling you with energy and life. Then open your eyes and return."

Encounter II

Wen was attentive and responsive to the guided imagery exercises, but over the long run the perception of her chest changed only minimally. The main change was noticeable immediately after treatment so we were challenged to make a greater and longer-lasting impact on the way she perceived her chest.

Goal

To further change Wen's chest image.

Guided Imagery

Exercise 1

> T guided Wen to allow the expansion of her chest to occur when lying in both positions: supine and side. She was instructed to imagine waves running through the body from the feet up through the

Cont'd...

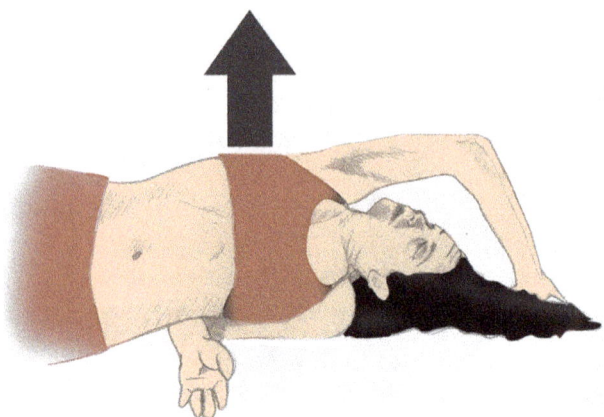

Fig. 5.18: While lying on her left side, Wen imagines a significant expansion of the right side of her chest.

Cont'd...

> *chest in front and on the sides. T told Wen to let the chest expand imaginatively to both sides of the room and in front, then come back to the normal limits of the body.*

Exercise 2

> *T asked Wen to compare her feelings and sensations on both sides of the chest and describe what she felt inside the lungs/chest and outside the body.*

Wen described that when she was lying on her left side and let the right lung and side of the body elongate toward the ceiling, her chest was expanding well, significantly more than when she lay on the right (Fig. 5.18). When she lay on the right side, her left chest moved up toward the ceiling to only half the extent that the other side did (Fig. 5.19). Then when asked to check the inside of the left chest she found beans and pebbles stuck inside the left chest.

Exercise 3

> *T instructed Wen to imagine holding a garden hose in her right hand and washing the beans and pebbles out through the left shoulder (Figs. 5.20A and B).*

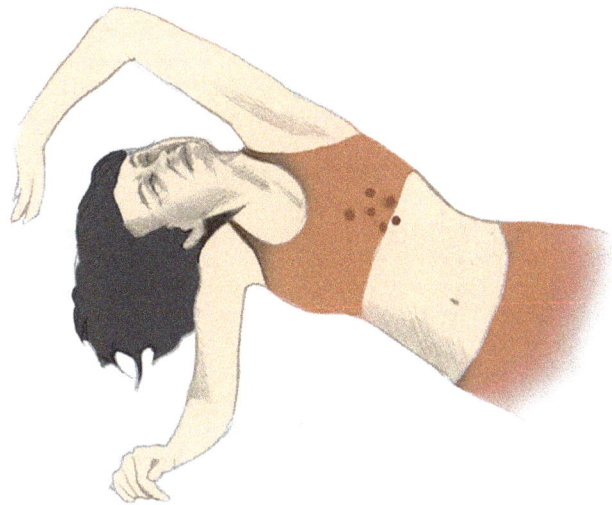

Fig. 5.19: While lying on the right side, Wen imagines limited expansion of the left side of her chest, with "beans and pebbles" inside.

Wen was able to remove the obstacle easily. The left chest became completely clear from within.

Wen described that she continued to feel better in terms of breathing with greater ease. After four months of therapy she rarely used her inhaler. Although she seldom used the inhaler, she still had difficulties perceiving the change in her asthma condition. At times, she felt very anxious and had the desire to grab the inhaler and use it, but once she utilized some of the guided imagery exercises, she felt no need for the inhaler. Wen was moving forward in the right direction but there was more work ahead to achieve further improvement.

Encounter III

T felt Wen needed to "face" her body, chest and posture. Facing meant for her being able to see herself in the mirror and alter what she saw for her own benefit. She practiced seeing herself and understanding what her desired posture and mobility were. It meant being able to mobilize the chest freely in all directions. Since Wen had a partial kyphotic (spine curved over in excess) upper body, all

94 *Moving Pain Away-RiVision®: An Innovative Physical Therapy Method*

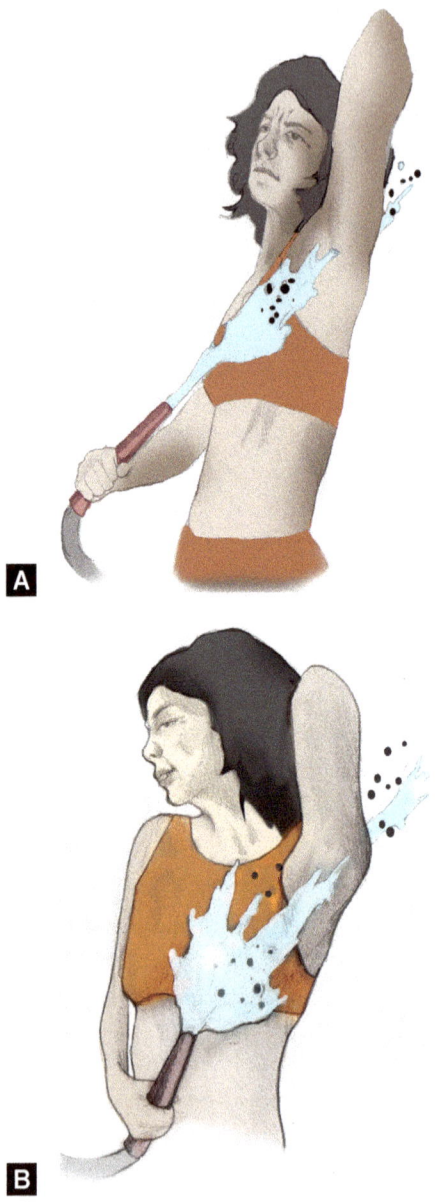

Figs. 5.20A and B: (A) Removing the obstacles; cleansing with the garden hose, side view, (B) Removing the obstacles; cleansing with the garden hose, front view.

therapeutic interventions were done gently while considering her physical limitation and inherent body structure. We practiced how to stand, sit and walk with more of an open chest, arm swings, and retracted shoulders while breathing with expansion. We spoke about the potential contributors to why she is so curved and sunk in the front of her chest. We explored body-mind connections with anecdotal confirmations. For example, Wen described being extremely anxious throughout life, recalling the way she was treated by her father. She revealed her father's abusive behavior toward the family as we progressed with the therapy (*see* encounter IV).

Goal

Heighten Wen's awareness of her chest to further enhance her ability to connect her chest status and her life experience.

Body Awareness and Dance/Movement Therapy

Exercise 1

> *Wen was encouraged to use all her body parts and to be more aware of them. T instructed Wen on specific chest, back and upper body exercises to warm up the tense area.*

Exercise 2

> T: *"Let the music touch and move inside the chest, back and forth, up and down and in circles while exercising the body (Fig. 5.21)."*

Wen stated that she never was able to experience her neck elongating up to the ceiling and this was her first time. Wen said, "It felt wonderful, moveable, soft and flexible. At the same time I can feel my feet and the top of my head, shoulders and arms. I felt connected! It was a wonderful new experience."

Guided Imagery

Wen reported that she felt more integrated versus feeling fragmented before starting this therapy. She described that her front chest was "like see-through glass."

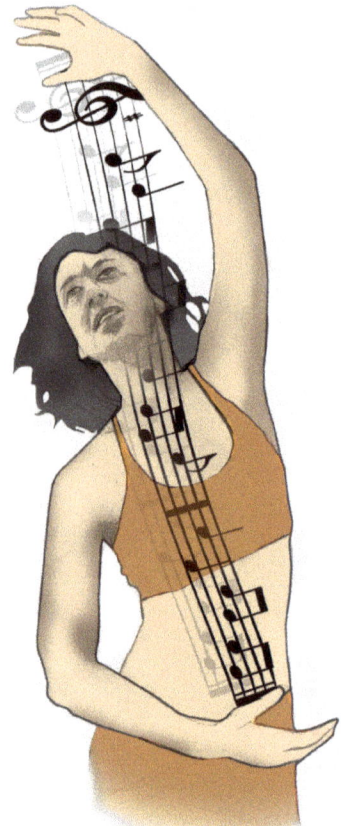

Fig. 5.21: Music moves inside Wen's body.

Exercise 1

T asked her to relate to the back of her chest, neck and head.

She could not feel them; as if they were not there. Guided imagery heightened her awareness of these parts. She was excited to be aware of more parts of the body.

Exercise 2

T guided Wen to imagine what her lungs looked like now after the guided imagery sessions.

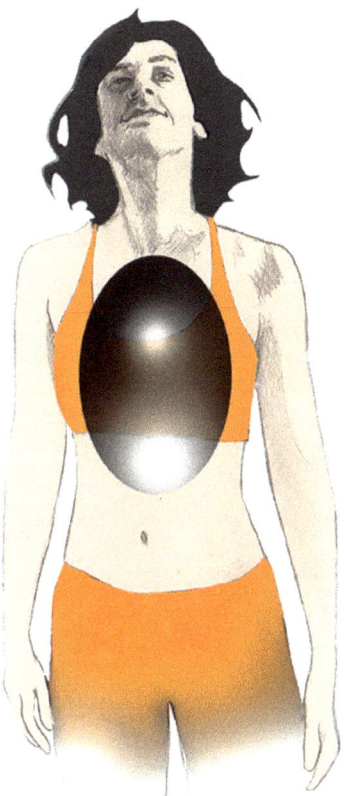

Fig. 5.22: Wen's chest area, clogged by an elliptical balloon.

She said that she saw the edges of her lungs colored rose-pink and very tight but the inside of the lung was envisioned as off-white, cream colored and more compliant. "My lungs feel like never before: more free, more present!"

> *T then added touch, which helped Wen to feel further at ease and less tense, and allowed her to imagine lighter colors.*

Encounter IV

Wen felt as though something was stuck in the lower part of her chest (base of diaphragmatic muscle) (Fig. 5.22). "This area is clogged with

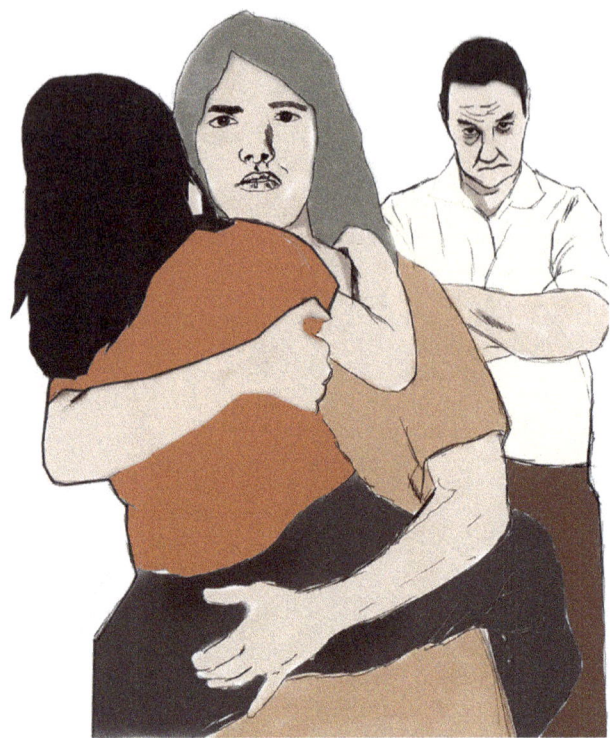

Fig. 5.23: Wen and her mom running away from her dad.

an elliptical balloon." Memories from childhood continued surfacing gradually. Wen allowed herself to revert (with T's assistance) to the time she could recall herself with her mom and dad. According to Wen, her dad was verbally abusive to them, shouting and threatening. Her mom was trying to protect her, holding Wen's small body. She remembered them running together out of the apartment to prevent her dad from hitting her mom (Fig. 5.23). She imagined seeing her upper body colored red and extremely tight.

Her father could not run after them fast enough since he was limping. They went to a relative's house and found solace with them. She further explained that logic should have propelled her mom to leave him, but in those times women did not leave their husbands, especially with young children to care for.

Then we regressed in time to a different occasion when she again experienced her chest as extremely tight and black. Her dad was intensely angry. At that time he was not getting help for his uncontrolled and dangerous outbursts of anger. Wen added, "So we were living in fear all the time for how and when he would strike us. He hit my mom several times but I do not recall him hitting my sister or me. This time we ran away to a relative's apartment and locked the door behind us. He was able to get to the apartment but was not able to open the door."

It was becoming highly possible that the more she was able to connect the external stimulus (traumatic family incidences) to her bodily sensations and feelings at that time, the greater positive release she would experience in the future. T encouraged her to be as descriptive as possible while providing a secure and supportive environment.

Goal

Connecting between severe childhood incidents and Wen's body sensations and feelings.

Guided Imagery

Following the session Wen was drained, so we energized the body with guided imagery exercises from Catherine Shainberg's book, *Kabbalah and the Power of Dreaming* (2005, pp. 26, 27).

Exercise 1

> *The Blue Vase*—"*Find a quiet place where you are not likely to be disturbed and where you can relax. Sit in an armchair with your arms and legs uncrossed. Close your eyes. Breathe out all that disturbs you, all that tires you, all that obscures you. Breathe it out as a light smoke (carbon dioxide) that is easily absorbed by the planet life around you. When your breath comes in on the inhalation, see it as blue as the radiant blue light from the sky, and filled with sunlight. See the blue golden light filling your nostrils, your mouth, your throat, and flowing down your back as a great*

Cont'd...

Cont'd...

> river of light. See it filling your feet, your toes, and stretching out of your toes as long antennas of light. See the light circulating up your legs to fill your pelvis, see it rising up into your chest, flowing in and out of your heart until your heart becomes a glowing blue lamp. See the light flow down your arms like smaller rivers of light, fill your palms and fingers, stretch out your fingers as long antennas of light. As you continue to breathe in the blue light, see the light continue to fill you. See it begin to radiate out of the articulations of your joints: out of your ankles, knees, hips, shoulders, elbows, and wrists. See the light fill you until it radiates out of your skin in all directions. See yourself as a crystal vase filled with light that radiates in all directions. Open your eyes, seeing yourself as a crystal vase radiating blue light in all directions. Then stop."

Exercise 2

> *The Pendulum*—"Close your eyes. Breathe out three times slowly, counting from three to one. Picture the number one as tall, clear, and bright. Imagine a great crystal pendulum rhythmically swinging from left to right, right to left. Each time the pendulum swings to the right, it gathers into a pile the (environmental) disruptions in your life which have caused a narrowing of your choices. Try to identify each disruption as the pendulum pushes it onto the pile. When all have been gathered, breathe out. See the pendulum swing wide to the right and swing back to the left in a great sweep, transporting the whole pile to the left. Breathe out and see the pendulum once again swing wide to the right and swing back to the left, knocking the whole pile off to the left and out of the picture. Breathe out and open your eyes."

Wen said that following the guided imagery exercises, her chest area, which had been painful before, was feeling significantly better. "I used to feel that I had a solidified ball stuck inside my chest. Now I feel that I want to crack this ball to pieces and get rid of it!"

Encounter V

Although Wen made substantial progress and needed her inhaler significantly less often than before, some of her days were better than others. After six months of steady improvement, Wen came to therapy one day experiencing extreme tightness in the chest and having a hard time coughing and breathing. She believed that her generalized anxiety, caring for her baby and other life stressors, were all contributing factors to the way she felt. Since she was breathing "from her shoulders," T noticed her shoulders moving up and down while the breath duration was relatively short. Light wheezing accompanied her breathing. Her chest and upper body were tight and stooped forward.

Goal

Reassure and remind Wen that she is equipped with PT, guided imagery and DMT exercises to utilize as needed.

Breathing Exercises

We practiced breathing exercises to adjust Wen's inefficient breathing pattern.

Exercise 1

> *T taught her to attain an appropriate sitting position while breathing: sit straight up with an open and expanded chest, working on expanding the ribcage in all directions. This could also be done while leaning on several pillows if Wen felt more comfortable that way. T added techniques to guide Wen's chest expansion.*

Once Wen was a bit calmer after a few sessions, T added guided imagery and DMT exercises. Our work was based on regular and continuous practice and exercises that Wen needed to do at home between sessions. Although she was willing to do so, life circumstances often distracted her from achieving her goal, yet she realized improvement as time went on (Figs. 5.24A and B).

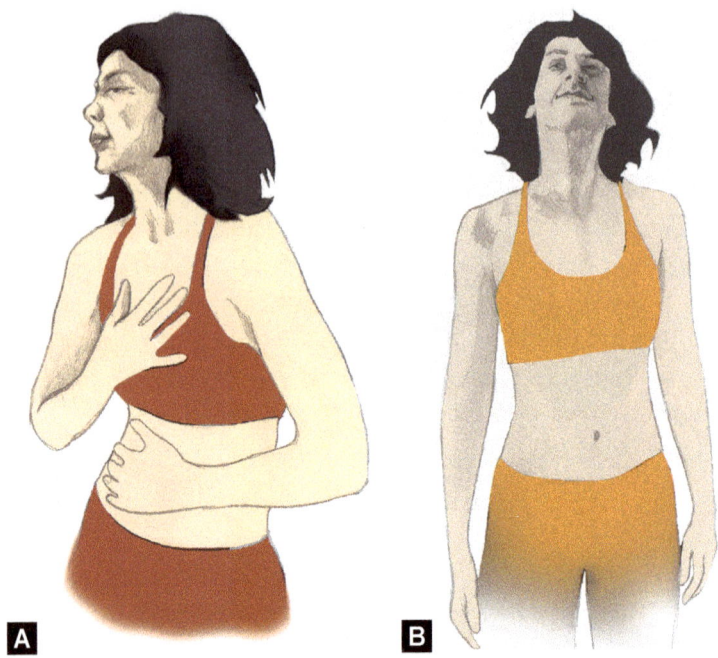

Figs. 5.24A and B: (A) Wen before treatment, (B) Wen after treatment.

CASE STUDY # 3—CHA

Cha was a pleasant, professional 38-year-old man residing in New York with hectic work schedule and a high-pressure job. He came to me complaining of severe, chronic neck and upper back pain, and stiffness that had lasted more than a year. He sought therapy for his neck from various medical doctors and physical therapists, but to no avail. The pain level had dropped a bit but was still a big hindrance to his everyday functioning. He told me that he did not want to be addicted to painkillers and was determined to assist himself on a more natural path.

We started therapy with the "conventional" physical therapy (PT) techniques: joint and soft tissue mobilization along with a prescribed home program of exercises. Although he was extremely busy and under a lot of pressure at work, he was eager to improve, was cooperative and attentive to the treatment approach and to my directives.

A physical evaluation revealed neck range of motion limitations, severe muscle stiffness and hypersensitivity to gentle touch. The pain radiated from the back and sides of the neck down to the shoulders on both sides and upper back. Following two months of the conventional PT approach, Cha described that he was improving minimally in terms of having less pain in the back of his neck; however, the stiffness in the affected area persisted.

At that stage I realized that incorporating guided imagery and DMT would benefit him by heightening his awareness of the connection between his neck condition and his tense life style.

GUIDE TO CHA'S TREATMENT

Encounter I

Around the end of the second month of his treatment, Therapist (T) realized that additional modes of therapy needed to be incorporated in order to further alleviate Cha's condition. T introduced him to guided imagery. He was open to listening and experimenting with it.

Goal

Enhance Cha's awareness of the connection between his neck condition and his tense life style.

Guided Imagery

Exercise 1

> T: "Allow yourself to feel and sense your body starting from the feet and going up all the way to the top of the head. Then, check if you are aware of all your body parts. Are all your body parts connected to each other?"

Cha described that he experienced his body as calm but his head is like a "stormy, windy blur." He further described imagining a tunnel from his mid-chest area up to the lower part of the neck. The head and the chest felt separated from each other since he could not imagine seeing the neck area (Fig. 5.25): "My neck piece is missing." Inside the tunnel there was some motion but the head was stiff and inert.

Exercise 2

> T prescribed breathing exercises to unlock the chest and rib cage area to allow a greater range of motion while Cha was sitting and lying down.

Cha continued to practice these exercises on a daily basis.

Exercise 3

> T instructed Cha to listen to relaxing music. Cha had played the piano in the past and loved classical music. T further instructed him to feel and sense the way his body responded to the music. "Now, check if the tunnel and head feel more connected, or how far apart you experience them from each other. Are they still separated or not?"

Cha stated that he was having a hard time with imagining the changes within his body while listening to the music.

Exercise 4

T tried to simplify the process by guiding Cha to use imagery as follows:

Case Studies: Treatment Goals, Exercises and Outcomes **105**

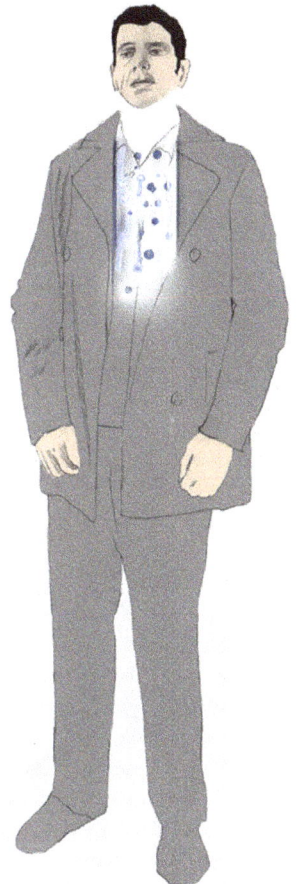

Fig. 5.25: Cha's initial body image—the neck is missing.

> T: *"Imagine movement through the tunnel being free and smooth in all directions: up and down, back and forth, and side to side."*

> T: *"Now imagine expanding the chest from side-to-side as far as it can go (Fig. 5.26)."*

Cha: "I am experiencing strong resistance to expanding."

> T: *"Imagine expanding the chest forward (Fig. 5.27)."*

Cha: "It is moving slightly."

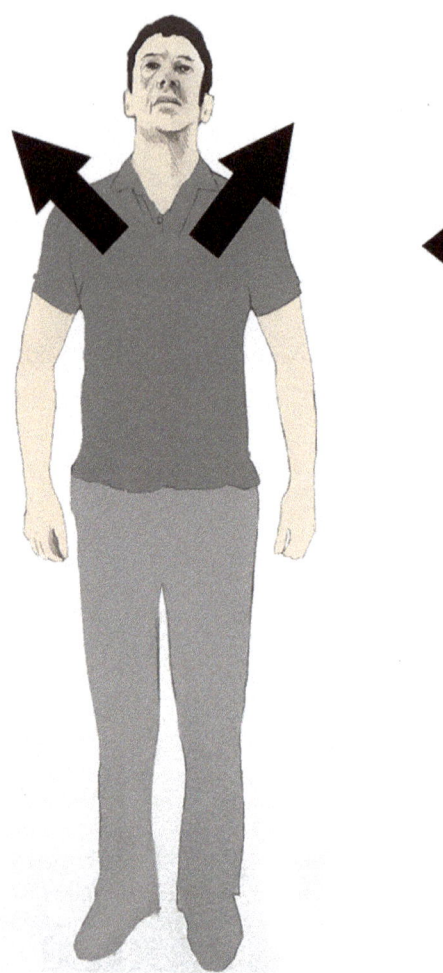
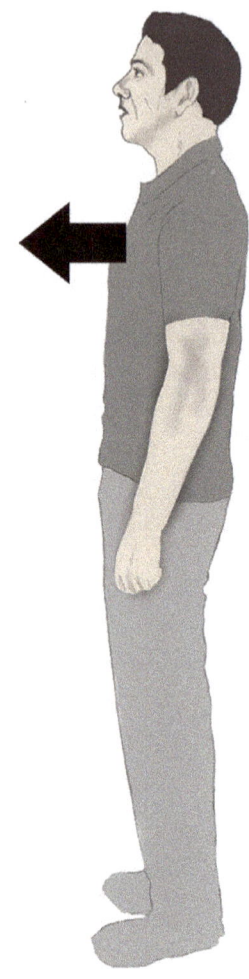

Fig. 5.26: Cha imagines expanding his chest sideways.

Fig. 5.27: Cha imagines expanding his chest forward.

T: *"Imagine expanding the chest backward (Fig. 5.28)."*

Cha: "There is almost no movement in this part."

T: *"Imagine elongating the top of the head toward the ceiling. What happens to your neck, chest and upper body?"*

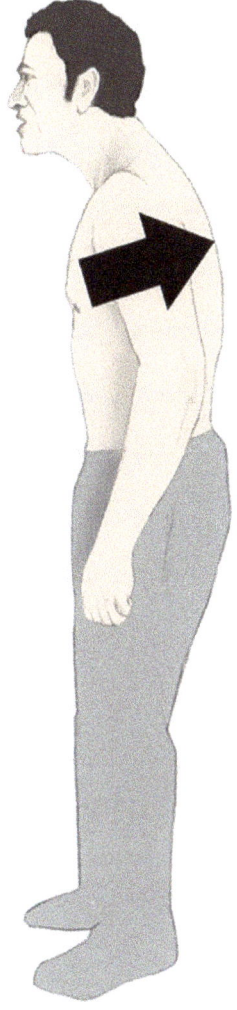

Fig. 5.28: Cha imagines expanding his chest backward.

Cha: "I can stretch somewhat and I feel release in the neck while doing so."

Goal

Enhance Cha's chest expansion capabilities.

Combining Dance/Movement Therapy and Guided Imagery

Exercise 1

> With background music, T encouraged Cha to use images of expansion to actually expand his chest, to feel as though he was occupying more space in the room, being more present.

Cha described that his chest still felt contracted and had a hard time expanding.

Exercise 2

> As we progressed in therapy, T asked Cha to evaluate and observe his encounters with people and what his chest "experienced."

For example, when speaking with Suzy, his good friend, Cha described his chest expanding to both sides as the amount of tension he felt decreased (Fig. 5.29). However, when he spoke with Christopher, a coworker who was hard to deal with, Cha felt his chest contract in pain while having a hard time breathing (Fig. 5.30).

> T instructed Cha to repeat this exercise for one month and make a list of the connections he found between external stimuli and his body's response.

During a guided imagery session the following month Cha described that at first, the more he tried to expand his chest in his imagination, the more resistance he experienced from "the tunnel" and inside his chest. As he continued the exercises, it got easier and both chest and "tunnel" responded in direct correlation (Fig. 5.31), meaning that when the chest expanded the tunnel widened as well.

Encounter II

Following eight weeks of therapy, we evaluated Cha's movement pattern and general ability to relate to his body. Although there had been a growing flexibility in the chest area, there was still something

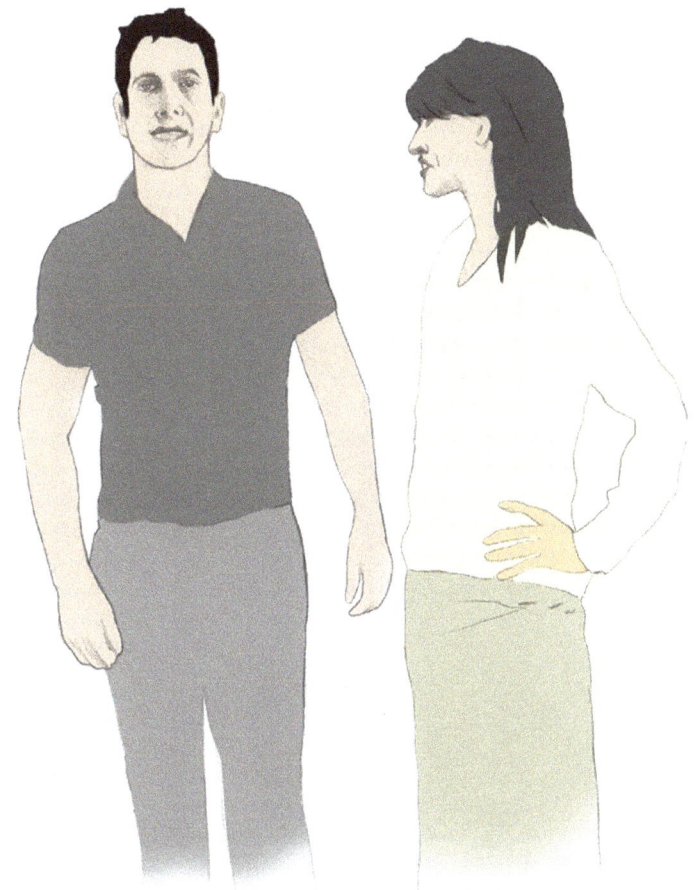

Fig. 5.29: Cha imagines interacting with Suzy.

inhibiting a full expansion. It was becoming clear to both T and Cha that his operating mode in everyday life relied heavily on his mind: logical reasoning dominated his functioning while his affect was minimal.

Goal

Try to lessen the "head as initiator" dominance and incorporate the heart and chest area more.

110 *Moving Pain Away-RiVision®: An Innovative Physical Therapy Method*

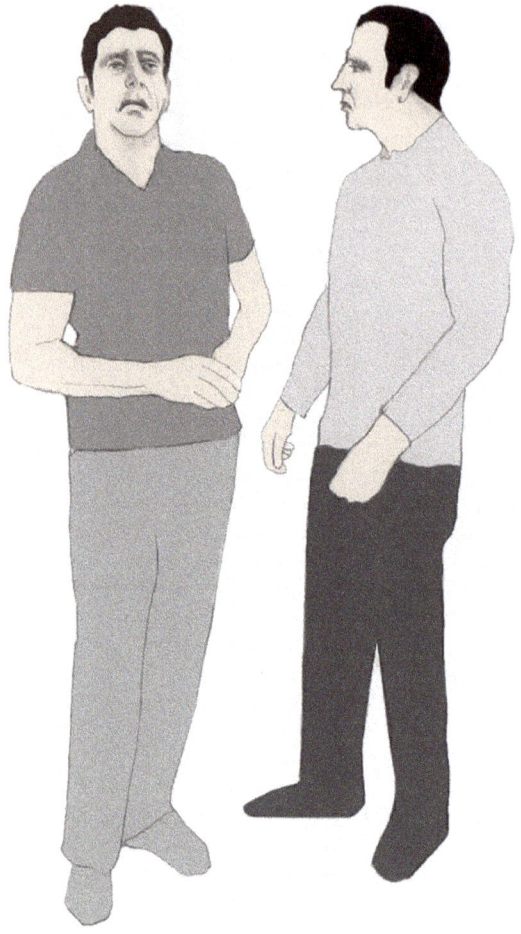

Fig. 5.30: Cha imagines interacting with Christopher.

Dance/Movement Therapy

Exercise 1

> *Concentrating on enlivening the "numb" chest area, T facilitated mobility of this area by asking Cha to touch his heart with the right hand and then with the left. Next T instructed him to touch his head with the right hand and then with the left. "What did you feel and sense in both experiences?"*

Case Studies: Treatment Goals, Exercises and Outcomes **111**

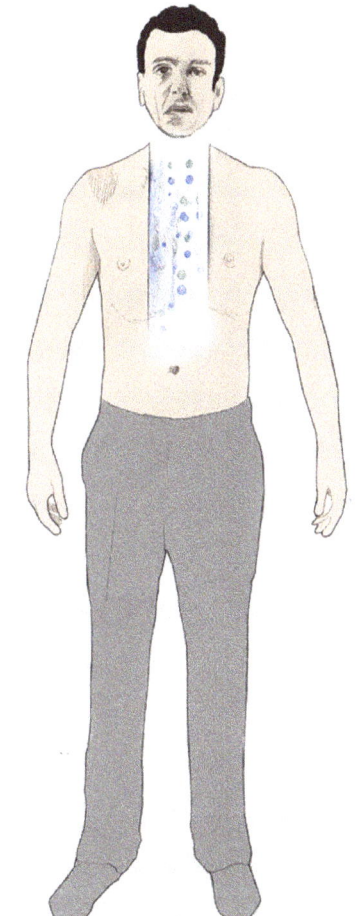

Fig. 5.31: Cha's chest and "tunnel" expand.

Cha responded that it was strange to touch the heart area since it was numb.

Exercise 2

> *T gave more exercises for the chest with and without self-touch. For example, bring chest in and out, and elongate and shorten the chest. Pretend that you are freezing or melting the chest and then breathe into different parts of the chest.*

Exercise 3

> T instructed Cha to massage his chest either with the help of his wife or by himself. The idea was that he needed to nourish and defrost this "frozen area."

Encounter III

At this stage Cha described that his chest was extremely vulnerable: "I am concerned that it will fall apart if I do more guided imagery and DMT exercises." He said that he imagined beams lying transversely inside his chest (Fig. 5.32). The sensation was so vivid to him that he could elaborate about the quality of the beams and the pins and screws that held them in place. The beams held the chest tightly and prevented any flexibility in this area. A large rod was situated where the neck was, though he was oblivious to the presence of his neck. His head was positioned above the rod and was disconnected from the chest.

Goal

Teach Cha to protect his vulnerable area.

Guided Imagery

Exercise 1

> T guided Cha to form an imaginative shield of light around the chest (Fig. 5.33): "Allow the golden shield to surround the entire chest when you need it."

Cha: "The shield makes me feel safer and stronger."

> T assigned homework: "Apply the imaginative shield before getting into tension-provoking situations. Take 20 seconds to put it in place and only then enter the room. Check what it does to you. How does it affect your chest, tunnel, head and neck?"

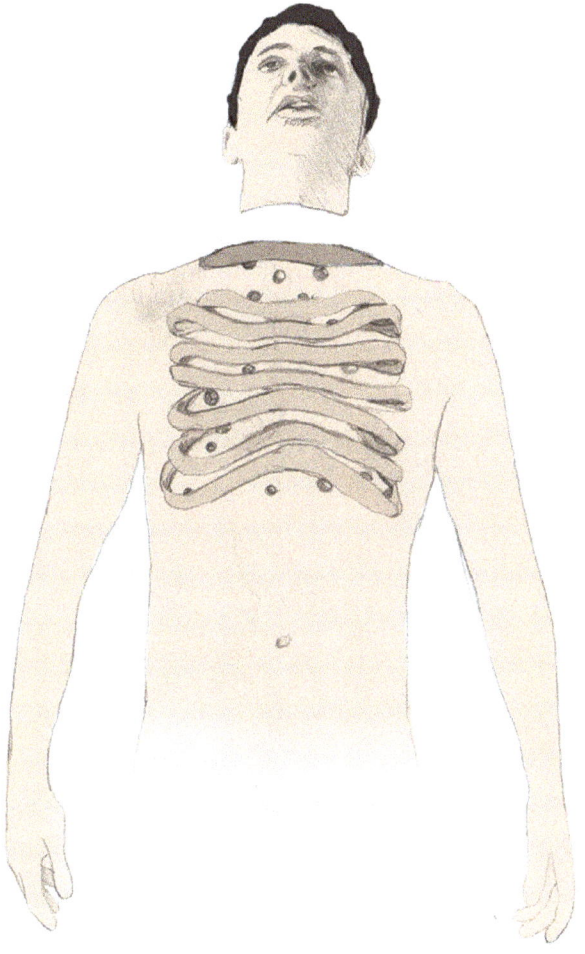

Fig. 5.32: Cha imagines beams inside his chest.

Exercise 2

> *T guided Cha how to practice simultaneously attending to his feelings and being logical in everyday life challenges, allowing his "feeling center" as well as his "head" to coordinate his responses to everyday life situations. "Practice feeling more when you encounter or converse with people."*

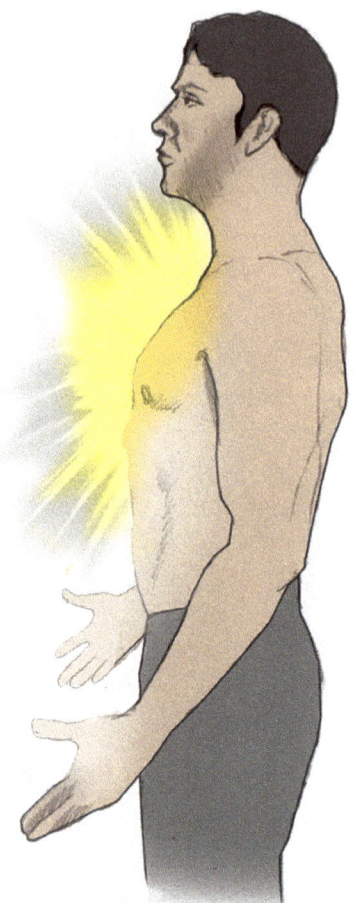

Fig. 5.33: Imaginative shield of light in front of Cha's chest.

Cha: "I have a hard time with this exercise. All that I do comes from my head while I block the feeling area."

Dance/Movement Therapy

Exercise 1

We practiced arm and hand movements, connecting head and heart areas in different anterior, posterior and lateral angles.

Upon re-evaluating Cha's neck condition he stated that his head felt calmer.

Cha: "When I stretch the top of my head, my neck lets go more than before. In addition, the image of the shield protects me well by preventing some of the tension in the chest."

Encounter IV

Although both Cha and T felt that he was starting to be able to perceive his chest with more motion, he continued to complain of tension and pain, although to lesser degrees.

Goal

To continue to warm up, nourish and revitalize the numb chest.

Guided Imagery

Exercise 1

> T guided Cha to invite the sun to hover above the center of the chest, pluck rays from the sun, position them in the center of the chest and see what happens. Then T told Cha to position the rays of the sun in different parts of the chest and evaluate.

Cha: "The chest feels looser and warmer. It is more alive."

Exercise 2

> T: *"Imagine presenting yourself in a meeting 'from the head' without talking. See if you can present yourself in a meeting 'from the chest' without talking."*

Cha responded that it took a great deal of effort to feel when he was concentrated on work-related issues and needed to cope with serious topics. His head was tense while his chest was still partially numb.

Dance/Movement Therapy and Guided Imagery

Exercise 1

> T: *"Exaggerate your chest motion in the DMT session and then eliminate your chest motions as much as you can. Experience the*

Cont'd...

Cont'd...

> vast difference in sensation and feeling when you engage the chest in opposite movements. Then stand and close your eyes, and imagine presenting yourself in a meeting 'from the head'—coldly, remotely, too cerebrally. And in comparison, present yourself in a meeting 'from the chest'—moving the chest to a great extent."

Cha described that he was more aware of his chest than before and could now feel more life and energy in his chest area when he imagined himself conversing with others in a meeting.

Encounter V

Cha's experience after three months of therapy was different than when we started. Initially, Cha experienced no motion between the chest and the head. Something was blocked inside the "tunnel" and the chest. He sensed dark small stones inside the "tunnel." After three months of treatment Cha revealed that "the tunnel" was less rigid, and there was a flow of movement between the "tunnel" and the head with moderate blockage only (Figs. 5.34 and 5.35). The flow was imagined as light blue watery material moving inside.

In the coming weeks Cha continued to describe a flow of warmth starting from the chest through the "tunnel" to the head with less of a hectic and stormy sensation in the head. He contributed a great deal of the improvement to the practice of the "protective shield." Following four months of therapy Cha described that the "rod" (that felt as if it was holding up his head) had disappeared for 95% of the time. The "tunnel" was soft and warm. The image of the beams inside and outside the rib cage disappeared and his pain level subsided significantly (90% less). Physical therapy evaluation revealed that the head motions of both extension and flexion were 80-85% better.

Cha's images had changed gradually as well. He could easily imagine forming the "shield" in front of his chest to feel more protected but he had a hard time visualizing it on the sides and back of the chest. In general, he felt emotionally stronger and courageous, allowing himself to contemplate the thought of changing jobs, where before he did not even consider it although he was not happy with what he was doing.

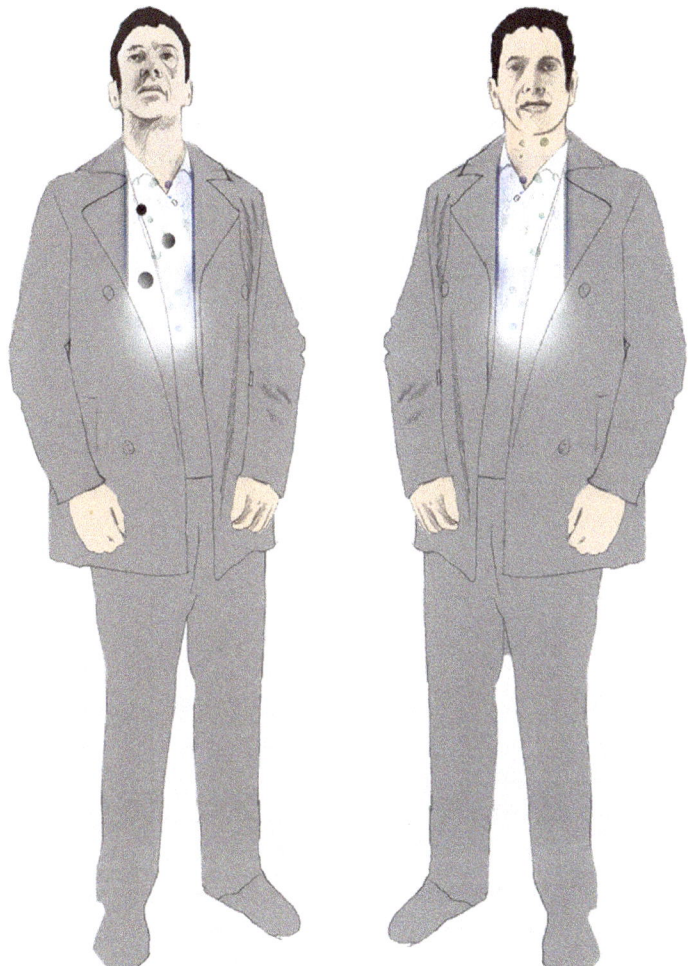

Fig. 5.34: Cha imagines moderate changes in his neck, chest and "tunnel".

Fig. 5.35: Cha imagines greater changes in his neck, chest and "tunnel".

Encounter VI

Cha described that as a lawyer who needed to deal with coworkers and clients, he felt only partially secure. Sometimes he felt as though his chest was getting smaller, he had some hard times breathing and he felt ignored by others when he presented his work. The amount of discomfort in the chest and body varied depending on the amount of stress and the number of people he encountered. The feeling that annoyed him the most was that he was not present strongly enough in the room while delivering his message or discussing relevant topics.

Goal

To enhance Cha's presence by "taking up more space."

Guided Imagery

Exercise 1

T guided Cha to imagine taking the elevator up to his office and checking out how much space he imagined occupying inside the elevator.

Cha: "I can barely see myself inside the elevator (Fig. 5.36). I feel as though I am almost not there. I possibly estimate occupying a square foot of the space."

T: "Now imagine entering an elevator in the building where you reside."

Cha: "I definitely take up more space but I am surprised that the space is still so minor, possibly 3 sq. feet of space."

T then asked Cha to practice growing inside the space using different directives. For example, "While in the elevator walk around it several times and feel the space around you. Then, pause."

Exercise 2

T asked Cha to find the actual center of the elevator and then to stand in this center with spaced out legs, forming a wide base of support. "Imagine with closed eyes that your space widens reaching both sides of the elevator. Imagine the ribs rubbing up against the sides of the elevator. Then let the body returns to its normal physical limits." Then T questioned Cha about how much space he imagined taking up from inside the elevator.

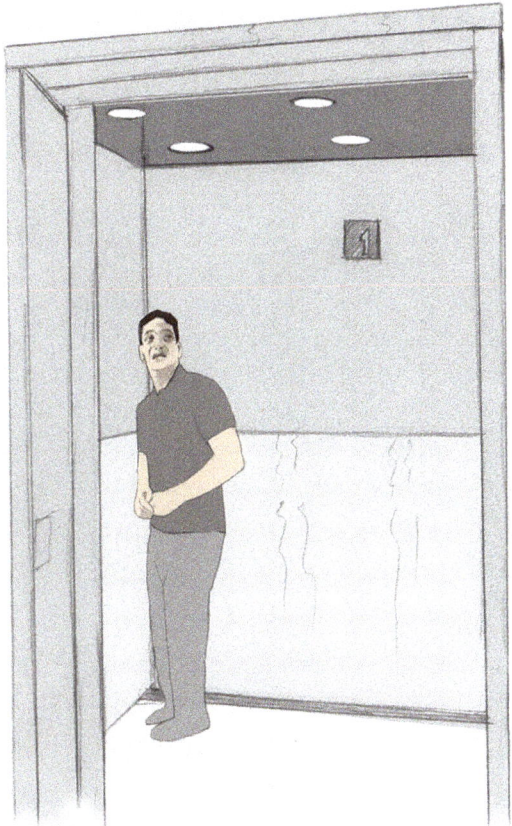

Fig. 5.36: Cha imagines occupying a small space in an elevator, feeling small.

Cha said that, at first, it was extremely artificial for him, but as time passed he was able to guide himself using T's directives and take up more space while feeling comfortable doing so. The guided imagery exercises, along with heightened body awareness and understanding that a change was needed, stimulated him to be vigilant about his home exercises.

Exercise 3

T encouraged Cha to compare the changes in his body when he is in tense and less tense environments.

> T: *"Check the difference between the enlargement processes happening at work and at home. Pay attention to what is blocking the expansion from inside. Why can't the body stretch out in your imagination?"*

Encounter VII

Cha was responding well to the guided imagery part of the treatment. However, T continued with the techniques to enhance his pace of improvement, particularly the amount of expansion in the chest area. Cha reported that he was feeling significantly better in terms of less pain in his neck and ability to move it more freely from one position to another. In addition, he could easily take up more room entering various spaces regardless of the amount of tension awaiting him. In addition, he felt that when he needed to negotiate sensitive, tension-provoking subjects with his clients, he had more confidence and an unfamiliar "new sense" of inner peace. He reported being stronger and more open to hearing and communicating with clients and coworkers.

Goal

Further the channels of communication with others by developing an open and larger chest image.

Body Awareness Exercises

Exercise 1

> *T gave Cha various assignments in which he was asked to chart what had happened to the size and shape of his chest when encountering particular people and situations.*

He did these for one month, then we explored and analyzed the connections between the external stimuli (person/situation) and his bodily changes. For instance, Cha described a client who used to give him a hard time at work. Each time he encountered this client he felt that his chest tightened, condensed and got smaller. He also had some slight breathing difficulties that brought about more tension. As in a vicious cycle, one thing propagated the other. T guided him to seek positive encounters and be aware of the difference between the negative and the more positive experiences in his body.

As time progressed, Cha described that he had an easier time sitting in meetings with his clients and coworkers, and presenting his arguments. He felt that he was not "talking from the head;" he felt that his chest was more present in the room as well as his whole body. The ideas he presented were "coming" from his upper body and not only from the head. He sensed warmth running up his chest all the way up to his head and imagined strong connections from his head down to the base of the chest. When entering a room he felt like a "big ship" entering an open space and occupying most of the empty space (Fig. 5.37). The pivotal point for him was that he felt that he radiated strength and was profoundly present.

Cha: "People approach me differently than before. It seems to me that it is easier to talk with me and get my responses. I am now more alive in my entire being and this propels people toward me more than ever before."

Guided Imagery

Exercise 1

> T: *"Imagine your arms and chest swinging from side-to-side forming a contralateral motion of the upper body on the lower body while walking, allowing the chest to rotate from side-to-side as you move forward."*

Cha was able to experience a change in his perception of his chest after the exercises. He could imagine swinging his arms and walking in a contralateral movement of upper body on lower body, taking up more space and feeling more present.

Exercise 2

> *Considering that before Cha started with the guided imagery exercises, he was not aware of his chest and neck, T then asked him to imagine more weight inside the chest while envisioning himself walking.*

Cha stated that he felt more grounded, his legs were planted better on the ground and he was aware of his chest more than before.

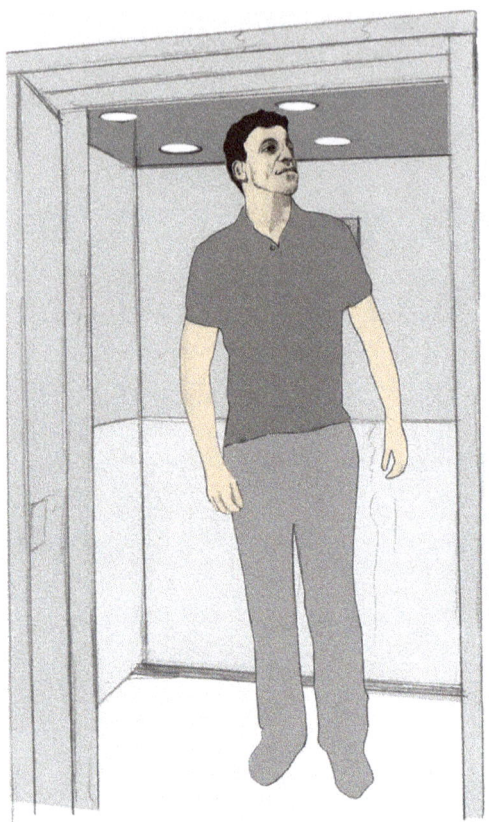

Fig. 5.37: Cha imagines occupying a large space in an elevator, feeling big.

Before therapy started Cha described that when he was arguing with a colleague his body would recede and he could not hold his space. Now, he was able to maintain his position literally without backing off or collapsing. His chest was strong and upfront. Although he was under constant pressure through work he experienced 95% improvement in pain level and stiffness.

After six months of treatment, once or twice a week, Cha was free of pain and stiffness. He was instructed to practice his home program exercises. At the 12-month follow-up, he described that he continued to improve and cope better in everyday life interactions related to his work.

CASE STUDY # 4—JANE

Jane was a 33-year-old secretary who came to treatment seeking help for a repetitive stress injury in her arms and shoulders that she had for the last year and a half. She stated that, "I have no power to keep myself up, I feel like I'm going to drop any minute (Fig. 5.38)." She was also diagnosed with tendinitis of her fourth and fifth fingers on both the right and left hands.

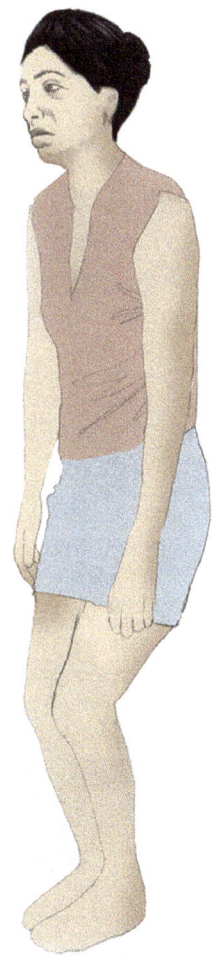

Fig. 5.38: Jane's posture before treatment.

Jane described that she used the computer a lot and as a result her pain worsened to the point that she could not use the computer more than five minutes at a time. In the mornings, she experienced numbness bilaterally at the fourth (ring) and fifth (pinky) fingers. Jane added that she had physical therapy (including ultrasound and therapeutic exercises) that did not help. She then got Lidocaine shots to her left forearm and cortisone shots to the right and left wrists, which did not help either.

Jane's upper body was profoundly slouched with a protruding neck and chin. Muscle strength evaluation revealed poor strength in both shoulders, elbows and hands. Her main complaint, in addition to the physical disorders we found, was that she felt she had no strength to hold her arms and upper body up. It sounded as though she was experiencing lack of energy in her upper body from the waist to the neck area. When I inquired about her ability to be strong and assertive in daily life encounters, she pointed out that she lacked assertiveness when she needed it and she felt fragile.

My assessment of Jane revealed repetitive stress injury to her shoulders, elbows and wrists along with poor posture and "inner stuff" that had to do with no energy in the upper body, an inability to assert herself, and her feeling extremely fragile.

GUIDE TO JANE'S TREATMENT

Encounter I

Jane was not aware of the fact that she was slouching forward in a significant way. She was, in fact, surprised to hear it. She had been concentrating on the weakness and the pain she felt. However, she never made a connection between her upper body shape and her shoulder, elbow, and hand conditions.

Goal

Heighten awareness of her posture.

Body Awareness Exercises

Exercise 1

> *Therapist (T) asked Jane to describe how she maintained her body in space. Then, T asked her to evaluate what the most comfortable posture for her was.*

Jane described that sitting and standing with a slouched upper body was the most comfortable position for her.

> *T then asked her to stay there and maintain the posture that she feels most comfortable attaining. After holding the "comfortable posture while being aware of it," T asked her to bring herself to the "opposite place"—sitting up erect, and evaluate what she sensed and felt.*

Jane described that it was very awkward to be in the erect posture, not at all comfortable and it seemed as if she was in an artificial place.

Exercise 2

> *T instructed Jane to return to where she felt was "the right" place for her body. T asked her to estimate how often during the day she was in this slouched posture and how often was she erect or partially erect.*

Jane responded that she estimated being upright maybe 10-15% of the time.

> *T then further recommended estimating her posture changes in the coming month by charting, on a daily basis, percentages of time she estimated attaining each posture.*

A few weeks later, Jane described that she was more aware of her postures now. She pointed out that the presence of another person also affected the way she held her body. For example, when speaking with her mom, whom she loved, she was partially erect and more open in her chest area (Fig. 5.39), but while speaking with her dad, from whom she was estranged, she slouched and experienced more weakness in the upper body (Fig. 5.40).

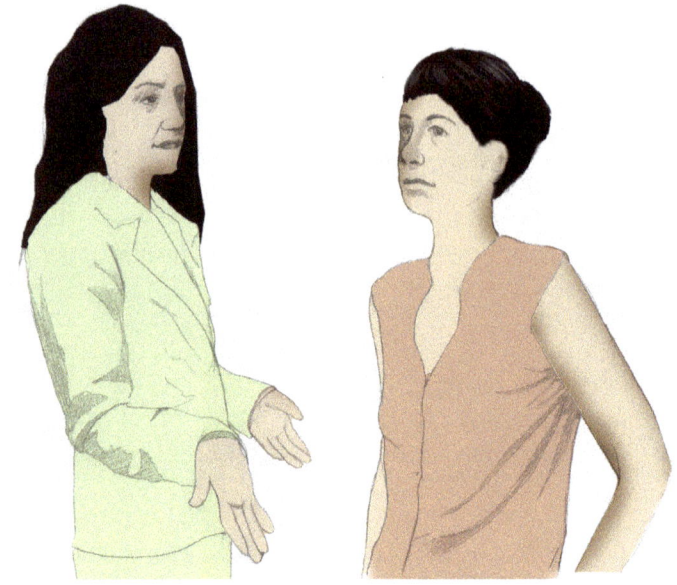

Fig. 5.39: Jane's posture around her mom.

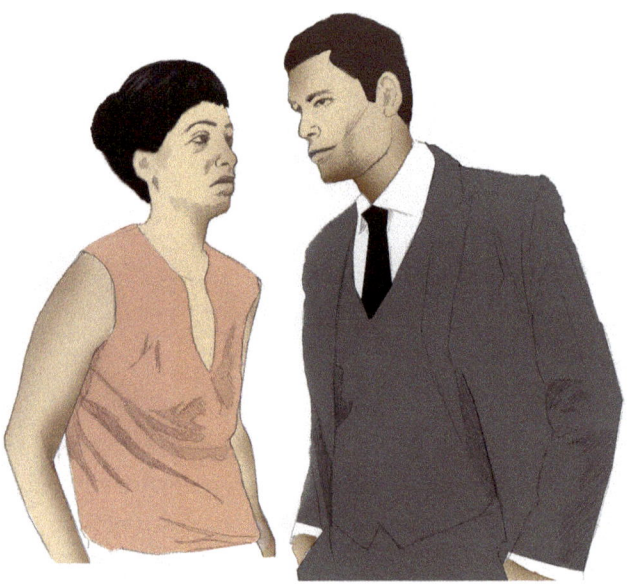

Fig. 5.40: Jane's posture around her dad.

Exercise 3

> T instructed Jane to further evaluate her posture when she talked to or met someone.
> T: *"Check when you tend to grow or shrink, get larger or smaller and become erect or bent over."*

Exercise 4

> T: *"Try to assume ¼ erect, ½ erect, ¾ erect positions. Can you do this? Check for four weeks."*

Exercise 5

> T: *"Check and observe your family and friends in terms of their posture. Make a chart of your findings."*

Jane came back with her information telling that her mother was fully slouched all the time, father was ¾ slouched 50% of the time, friends Jim, Tom and Chris were ¾ slouched 70% of the time.

> T: *"Why is it that your friends are slouched to a noticeable amount? Is there a common denominator between your postures? What do you get from their postures that resemble yours? What kind of emotion or attitude is connected with their postures? Continue to observe yourself and others."*

Exercise 6

> T asked Jane to observe and acknowledge under which conditions or situations she was able to assume more of an erect posture. That is, when in front of many people? When with her closest friend? Under which conditions or situations did she tend to slouch farther?

Jane thought that her posture provided her with protection from perceived threats from people or situations she encountered.

Goal

How to change posture but stay protected.

Guided Imagery

Exercise 1

> T: *"Imagine someone pushing you strongly, trying to push you down. How do you protect yourself from falling? How can you protect your chest? Imagine someone pushing you from the front backward. How can you protect the front part of your chest? Then, imagine someone pushing you from behind forward or sideways. How can you protect your chest in each direction?"*

Exercise 2

> T: *"Imagine someone pushing your heart area. How can you protect your heart area?"*

Jane was trying to experiment with the different images T introduced. She was struck by the lack of energy she experienced in her upper body. She compared her upper body to a rag-doll body with no bones or firmness, susceptible to collapsing at any given time (Fig. 5.41). The ability to protect her chest was foreign to her.

Goal

Develop awareness of the emotion-chest relationship.

Guided Imagery

Exercise 1

> T: *"During daily activities allow yourself to evaluate what image you set around your chest when:*
> - *Someone puts mental pressure on you.*
> - *Someone comforts or loves you.*
> - *Someone argues with you.*
> - *Someone ignores you.*
>
> *Based on the circumstances above, pay attention to which body part(s) and emotion(s) are evoked."*

Jane said: "When I am relaxed my chest is wider and softer. I have a light blue color surrounding my chest. When I am tense, my neck

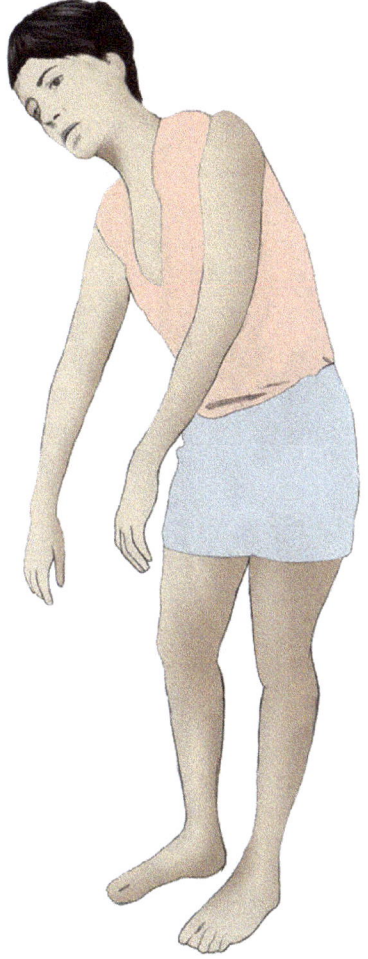

Fig. 5.41: Jane's rag-doll body image.

gets very tight like I have fire going up and down my neck. When I am discouraged by circumstances, I get weaker, smaller, and sit more slouched."

Exercise 2

T was trying to help Jane notice what would happen when pleasant and unpleasant objects were applied around her chest.

> T instructed Jane to imagine "protective material," like cotton, and "non-protective material," like sharp toothpicks, being in contact with her chest.
> T: "Imagine what happens to your chest when soft and harsh stimuli are around it. How do you cope with it?"

Jane described that when she imagined having a strong unpleasant sensation around her chest she started running away: "I am removing myself from the situation."

Encounter II

It was clear to both Jane and T that Jane had a hard time perceiving what was happening on a bodily level in her chest/upper body. Although she wanted to feel better, she was only at the initial stage of experiencing and feeling her chest/upper body. Utilizing imagery work was of great interest to her, but she had difficulties in fully connecting between her body posture and her physical manifestations. At this stage of the work she said that since she had a narrow chest that did not want to be fully present, obvious and known to others, the imagery exercises were cumbersome to perform.

Based on her feedback, T recommended more basic exercises as described below.

Goal

Use simple directives to enhance the correlations between body-posture and emotion.

Body Awareness Exercises

Exercise 1

> T: "Why do you sit slouched? What does it do for you? Do you want to change it now? Can a change in your posture make you feel more comfortable inside? Can you change your posture without feeling comfortable?"

Exercise 2

> "If you try to make a change gradually from inside, what do you feel and sense?"

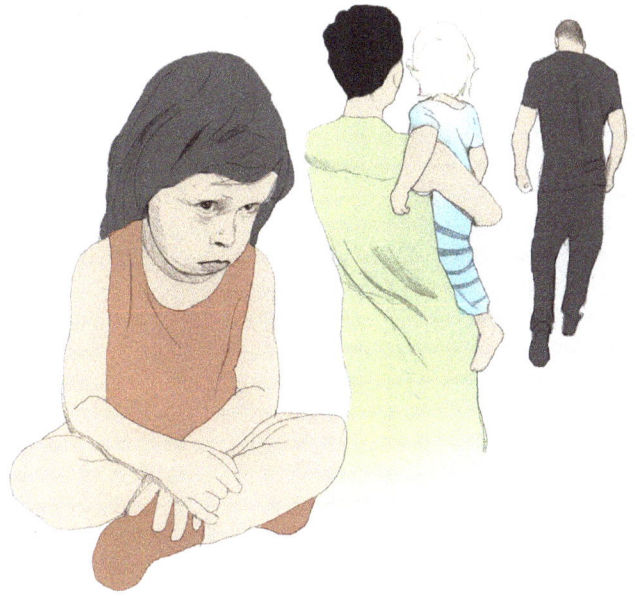

Fig. 5.42: Jane's father leaves his family.

Exercise 3

> *"If you try to make a change forcefully from inside, what happens?"*

Jane: "My father left us at a young age—he did not want me (Fig. 5.42)." She added that she had low self-esteem and did not want to be noticed by others. Something in her felt that she was not worthy enough because her father did not want her. She continued saying that her back, neck and shoulder musculature were too weak. She believed that she probably did not have the strength to be by herself and would need some help to overcome hurdles in her life.

Breathing Exercises

T incorporated breathing exercises that are often practiced in physical therapy. Jane liked these exercises and said they helped a bit. Then T incorporated breathing exercises along with movement and music emphasizing expansion, contraction and side-to-side movements of the chest area. T asked her the following:

Exercise 1

> "While breathing, check whether the air is flowing to the entire chest or not and, if not, which parts are deprived of air according to your perception?"

Exercise 2

> "Which parts of the chest/rib cage are moving fully, partially or not moving at all?"

Exercise 3

> "Following the breathing exercises, with or without the music, evaluate what has changed in the way you feel and sense this region."

Goal

Observe movement patterns in dance/movement (DMT) sessions in relation to the chest area.

Dance/Movement Therapy

Exercise 1

> T asked Jane to check how the chest, shoulders, and neck were involved in the movement itself, looking for patterns.

Jane described that she moved her shoulders when she needed to erect her spine with minimal opening and expansion from the front of her chest. As a result, the shoulders were more involved in being upright than her chest and rib cage areas.

Encounter III

Jane elaborated on the feelings she experienced when she attempted to be erect: "The entire upper body is so fragile that being upright requires extra powers which I believe I am lacking."

Goal

Reinforce Jane's attempts to erect her spine while coming out of her comfort posture.

Body Awareness and Physical Exercises

Exercise 1

> *T asked Jane which movements she could not do or had a hard time doing. T continued by asking Jane to stay within these hard motions and feel and sense herself.*

For example, Jane described that she had the most difficulty fully erecting her spine: "I am going to collapse any minute. It is too hard for me. It makes me take up too much space and be too present. People can notice me!"

Exercise 2

> *T allowed Jane to relax and check how she felt. T introduced the erect positions by practicing them in a more gradual manner: beginning from going up a quarter of the way, to half way, to all the way upright, all the while evaluating how she felt and sensed her body while changing the extent of spine erection.*

Exercise 3

> *T asked Jane to find her center of being, her weak and strong areas, which body part pulls her down, and which body part can potentially lift her up (Figs. 5.43A to C).*

Goal

Try to identify the core of the problem—where the fear of being upright and present is coming from.

Body Awareness Exercises

Exercise 1

> *Since Jane repeatedly stated: "I hate taking up space. I hate showing power and I dislike being so present," T asked her various questions trying to explore why she felt this way. "What triggered it?"*

Jane wanted to talk and share her past, she needed to be heard but the exploration process was slow and painful. After a while, she elaborated that her father had left her mother, her sister and herself,

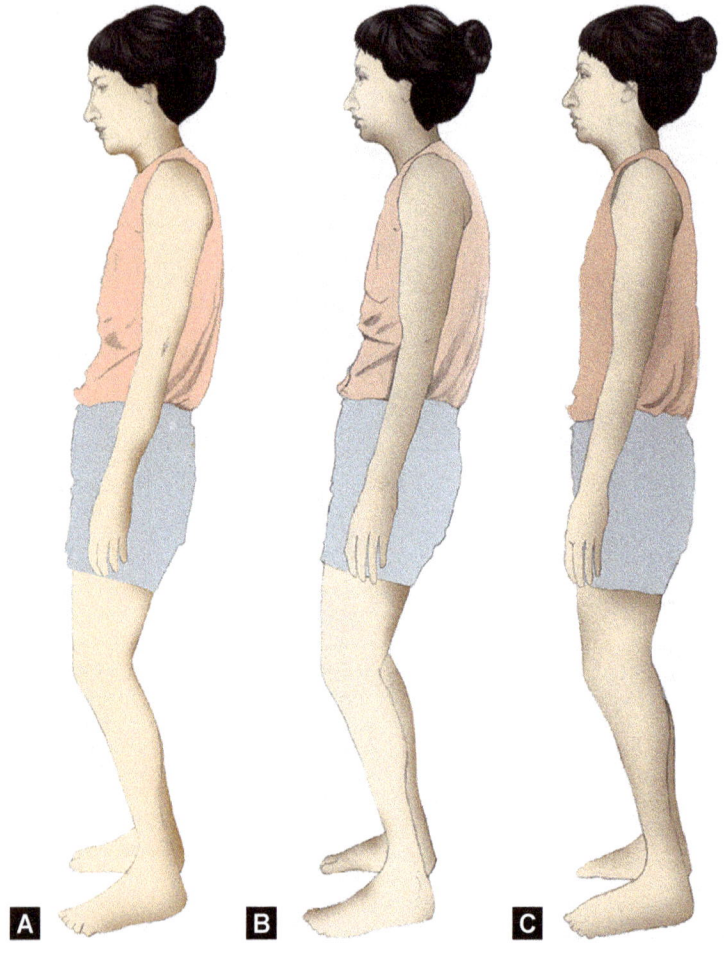

Figs. 5.43A to C: (A) Jane's posture before treatment, (B) Jane's during treatment, (C) Jane's improved posture.

and only by being not noticed could she cope with his behavior. Only by feeling that no one needed to see her (in a way, she was disappearing from sight) could she survive his departure.

> *T continued to encourage Jane to make the connection between her posture and this past incident which led her to want to disappear from view.*

Jane made a very distinct connection: "When my dad was around, I always needed to be small, ceasing to exist in the room."

SUMMARY

In this chapter, four case studies detailed patients' stories and their course of treatment. Each case study described treatment goals and a range of effective exercises tailored to achieve them.

Chapter 6

Apply the RiVision® Method

How can you apply the information presented in this book to your needs? You may be in the process of trying different treatment protocols because you are experiencing chronic pain. Or, you may be curious to know more about alternative treatment options because you or someone you know may need a multidimensional treatment approach to better their condition.

FINDING THE "REPETITIVE STRESS PATTERN"

At the very first stage of the treatment, you will try to identify the "Repetitive Stress Pattern" (RSP) that may have led to your chronic pain or musculoskeletal disorder. RSP is the negative prolonged, repetitive event that affects you emotionally and physically.

RSP is similar in many respects to "Repetitive Stress Injury" (RSI)—a physical condition characterized by damage to tendons, nerves and soft tissues, usually affecting people who habitually perform repetitive motions over a prolonged period of time (American Heritage Medical Dictionary, 2007).

While RSI relates to the mechanics, body alignment and awkwardness of the joint position, RSP (when taken into account during RiVision®) also addresses the prolonged stress upon the mind. RiVision® addresses the impact of long-term repetitive reactions to stressful situations on feelings and sensations inside and outside your body, as well as your typical body motions. The cause-effect relations are summarized in Table 6.1.

As you read the book, please refer to the "Reader Response" section in Chapter 4. This section requires that you answer questions. There are no right or wrong answers and your responses should reflect your experience. Some therapeutic exercises are more relevant

Table 6.1: Event/Interaction-Feelings-Sensations-Typical Motion Factors—Use of Planes

Event	Feelings (emotions)	Sensations (physical)	Typical motion factors	Use of planes estimated in percentages
			Firm/Fine scale: 0–10	Horizontal (side-to-side motions):
			Sudden/Sustained scale: 0–10	Vertical (up and down motions):
			Direct/Indirect scale: 0–10	Sagittal (back and forth motions):
			Free/Bound Flow scale: 0–10	

to you than others and you should concentrate on them. The more precise you are in terms of your feelings and sensations, the better equipped you will be to practice this method.

CHARTING YOUR RESPONSES

Before charting your responses, review the following example of a patient's response to the exercises. This will assist you in charting your own responses. The patient described her experience of muscle tension manifesting in two different environments: hostile and pleasant.

After the patient completed the two tables (two different environments for events of: initial response; after 1 month; after 2 months) she was able to compare the results to find common denominators and repeated patterns. She chose the following set of exercises related to muscle tension motion factors, described earlier in Chapter 4.

- Relate to the level of free flow on a scale from zero to ten where zero is completely free flow and ten is an extreme bound flow. How would you define your "body state" on this Free/Bound Flow Scale?
- Practice motions that begin free and become increasingly bound. Then move in the opposite direction, from bound movements to free.

- Think of a person you know who demonstrates either extreme rigidity or extreme softness in movement.
- How do you perceive yourself on the Free/Bound Flow Scale: at work, in tense situations, at home?

Example of Patient's Response to a Hostile Environment

> *Event*: Several coworkers are extremely critical of her work's performance.

Feelings: She feels that others dislike her and criticize her most of the time; she becomes moderately anxious.

Sensations: "My arms and hands are loose and lack energy. They feel weak. However, I experience my middle body region, especially my pelvic and abdominal regions, as tight, bound, painful, and ice-like."

Typical motion factors: "My arms and hands move freely, possibly three to four on the Free/Bound Flow Scale. However, when trying to move my middle body region, it feels tight and bound, possibly seven on the Free/Bound Flow Scale."

Use of planes: She described using the downward motions of the vertical plane 60% of the time, the horizontal plane 30%, and the sagittal plane 10% of the time (*see* Fig. 4.1).

The patient then summarized her experiences in Table 6.2 (initial encounter, 1 and 2 months after initial encounter).

Example of Patient's Response to a Pleasant Environment

> *Event*: My boyfriend and his family love and accept me.

Feelings: I feel relaxed and secure 80% of the time.

Sensations: "My arms and hands feel normal in terms of strength and energy level. In a pleasant environment there is less discrepancy between the way I experience my arms and my middle body compared to an environment of hostility. My arms are more 'alive' and my pelvis is less tight."

Typical motion factors: She described that in a pleasant environment there is a smaller difference in the free-bound flow between

Table 6.2: Experience of Hostile Environment.

	Feelings being disliked and criticized by others	Sensations	Typical motion factor Free/Bound flow scale 0–10	Use of planes estimated in percentages		
				Horizontal (side-to-side motion)	Vertical (up and down motion)	Sagittal (back and forth motion)
Initial encounter	90% of the time	Arms and hands lack energy and are weak. Middle body region (pelvis and abdomen) is tight, rigid and painful	Pelvis 7 Arms 3	30%	60% downward motion	10%
1 month after	80% of the time	Same as initial encounter	Pelvis 8 Arms 3	25%	65% downward motion	10%
2 months after	75% of the time	Same as initial encounter	Pelvis 6 Arms 4	25%	60% downward motion	15%

her arms and her middle body area; the muscle flow is more balanced in both areas (five on the Free/Bound Flow Scale).

Use of planes: She described using the downward motion of the vertical plane 50% of the time, the horizontal plane 40%, and the sagittal plane 10% of the time (*see* Fig. 4.1).

The patient then summarized her experiences in Table 6.3 (initial encounter, 1 and 2 months after initial encounter) and compared them.

ANALYZING THE PATIENT'S RESPONSES

The patient was able to define and grade the repeated cause-effect patterns of movement based on her answers in Tables 6.2 and 6.3. Here are some findings:

When she experienced hostility, her pelvis was more bound (six to eight on the Free/Bound Flow Scale) and her arms had a more free flow (three to four on the Free/Bound Flow Scale) compared to the flow in a pleasant environment. When in a pleasant environment, she was in the mid-range (five on the Free/Bound Flow Scale) in all three evaluations of her arms, hands, and pelvis. She used the downward motion in the vertical plane more often than the horizontal and sagittal planes in both hostile and pleasant environments; however, the use of the downward vertical planes was more pronounced when in a hostile than in a pleasant environment.

The information gathered by the patient can highlight the potential cause-effect patterns that may lead to chronic pain. In this case, the downward prominent posture of the spine along with the tight pelvis may be causing the chronic back pain. At this stage the reader may be able to understand the cause-effect relations and to realize the impact on her ability to achieve a better outcome (at this point, you may be able to use part of the method independently. However, to undergo the in-depth treatment of RiVision® you will need to consult with the practitioner). Monitoring over time allows the patient to see more clearly her repeated patterns.

HOW TO UTILIZE RIVISION®

Based on the examples outlined above and your own response to the exercises, you should be able to determine what you have learned

Table 6.3: Experience of Pleasant Environment.

			Typical motion factor	Use of planes estimated in percentages		
	Feelings being relaxed and secure	Sensations	Free/Bound flow scale 0–10	Horizontal (side-to-side motion)	Vertical (up and down motion)	Sagittal (back and forth motion)
Initial encounter	80% of the time	Arms/hands are more "alive" and pelvis less tight when comparing to the experience of Hostility (see Table 6.2)	Pelvis 5 Arms 5	40%	50% downward motion	10%
1 month after	75% of the time	Same as initial encounter	Pelvis 5 Arms 5	35%	55% downward motion	10%
2 months after	85% of the time	Same as initial encounter	Pelvis 5 Arms 5	35%	50% downward motion	15%

with RiVision® and how to apply it. This will positively affect your musculoskeletal condition and pain level. It has been my experience that after acquiring greater experience and awareness, patients are able to determine the cause-effect relations resulting in significant improvement in their symptoms. One patient reported that after being aware of the cause-effect relation between the way she felt around her demanding mother and her tense back, her back pain subsided. She believed that after following the recommended exercises (*see* Chapter 4) and identifying each of the elements (event, feelings, sensations, typical motion factors and the use of planes), she clearly understood her RSP and could let go of the back tension.

Other patients required a larger period of time (months) to understand and experience the cause-effect relations before acknowledging a positive change. They attest to the fact that perseverance played a significant role in attaining the desired results after they were enrolled in an active, more in-depth, body-mind role. Unlike conventional physical therapy, patients and therapists practicing RiVision® are asked to have a greater insight into their own body-mind weaknesses, encouraging them early in their treatment course to unravel the cause-effect relations and their physical manifestations.

Chapter 7

Summary

The ability to change a pattern and find a new form of moving and feeling comes once you have developed enough awareness of where you are "stuck," or what your particular patterns are. The attachments you develop toward your movement patterns have a significant meaning: they serve to protect you. Your movement patterns can be present for many years without being changed. Many people live well using the same, idiosyncratic patterns without being motivated to change them. Several reasons can explain why we do not have the motivation to change. People may have lived in peace with their movement patterns and themselves or may not have been aware of their specific movement style. Others may not be conscious of the fact that the body and mind can strongly impact each other and that change in one aspect can affect the other in a positive manner.

Our style of movement can serve us well, as long as we do not suffer physically or emotionally from our body. However, once our body is compromised we start considering treatment and modifications of our old negative habits.

The process of going through these renovations requires a state of readiness and openness. It requires a clear intention regarding what needs to be altered in order to function better in everyday life. It goes hand-in-hand with feeling and negotiating life better.

Notice if you can trace which emotions and motions *you* are "stuck with." In other words, which emotions and motions do you repeat more than you think you should? Which postures, gestures, or facial expressions are too dominant for your well-being (i.e., you do them in excess and, therefore, they may be inappropriate and exhausting to you and your surroundings)? Consider an architectural metaphor: If the beams in your house are not placed well to hold the weight of the house (e.g., too many beams on one side versus the other side of the house), the entire house will be out of balance. So the intention is to use balanced elements to maintain an integrated, strong architectural persona.

The range of the change in a pattern is up to us and can be altered in various ways. It can affect our self-acceptance, self-control, and comfort level inside our body and mind. Therapists and patients need to recognize that, when trying to cope with chronic pain, conventional physical therapy may not suffice. Despite the idea that there are psychological benefits to physical therapy, this therapy does not address the subconscious process involved in chronic pain. I found that the simultaneous usage of physical exercises and modalities relating to the subconscious is superior to the sole usage of physical training when treating pain and mood.

The goal of the Chace technique of dance/movement therapy (DMT), which uses dance as the medium of expression, is to enhance the individual's capacity for emotional release, while increasing awareness of movement preferences and intentions (Levy, 1988). This treatment entails physical activity and also evokes the subconscious processes. In this technique, the subconscious is explored, among other things, through imagery, in which the therapist offers an image which resembles the person's movement pattern so the patients can be more in tune with the subconscious material of their being (Levy, 1995). Wright and Mischel (1982) used a modified version of the Mood Adjective Check List and found that imagery alters emotional states. Imagery of happy events led to positive feelings and imagery of sad events led to negative feelings. Imagery utilized in DMT and guided imagery elicits such subconscious feelings.

The usage of DMT and guided imagery as well as various physical therapy modalities form the basis of the RiVision® method. RiVision® offers the reader an innovative, multidimensional way of evaluating and treating chronic pain and musculoskeletal disorders. Unlike other physical therapy treatments that deal with chronic physical pain and musculoskeletal disorders, RiVision® simultaneously relates to a large array of physical and emotional manifestations of pain. Patients and therapists practicing this method are encouraged to develop a greater awareness of their body-mind weaknesses from an early stage of the treatment by identifying the "Repetitive Stress Pattern" that may have led to their chronic pain.

RiVision® consists of elements within physical therapy, DMT, and guided imagery practice. In physical therapy, it relates to a patient's range of motion, pain level, posture and function levels. In DMT, it relates to a patient's usage of the vertical, horizontal and sagittal planes of motion as well as the general typical pattern of movement. In guided imagery, RiVision® relates to the images the person describes inside and outside her body in relationship to daily encounters with other people and events.

The art of integrating various modalities incorporated within RiVision® that will best fit the patient's needs is of great importance. To accomplish the desired outcome, it is recommended that the treatment method be specifically tailored to each patient by following one of seven protocols of treatment outlined in this book.

Bibliography

Action-Profile Review. Denver, Colorado: Action Profilers International, Ltd.; Fall, 1988.

Andrade CK, Clifford P. Outcome-Based Massage, 2nd edition. Baltimore, MD: Lippincott Willimas & Wilkins; 2008.

Chaiklin S, Schmais C. The Chase approach to dance therapy. In: Sandel SL, Chaklin S, Lohn A (Eds). Foundation of Dance/Movement Therapy: The life and Work of Marian Chace. Columbia, MD: The Marian Chace Movement Fund of the American Dance Therapy Association; 1993. pp. 75-97.

Chapman RC. Chronic pain syndromes of psychologic/psychosocial origin—introduction. In: Bonica JJ, Loeser JD, Chapman RC, Fordyce WE (Eds). The Management of Pain. Malvern, PA: Lea & Febiger; 1990. pp. 284-6.

Feldenkrais M. Awareness through Movement: Easy-To-Do Health Exercises to Improve Your Posture, Vision, Imagination, and Personal Awareness. San Francisco: Harper Press; 1990.

Har-El Belach R. The psychological implications of moving in different planes. Master Thesis. New York: Hunter College; 1991.

Har-El Belach R. Influence of neck exercises, combined with either the chance technique of dance therapy or aerobic training, on pain perception, mood state, and cervical range of motion of adults with chronic mechanical neck pain. Doctoral Dissertation, New York University. 2000.

Har-El Belach R. (2016). Author's website www.drrivi.com.

Knaster M. Discover the Body's Wisdom. New York: Bantam Books; 1996.

Kraus R, Hilsendanger SC, Dixon B. History of the Dance in Art and Education, 3rd edition. Englewood Cliffs, NJ: Prentice-Hall, Inc.; 1991.

Laban, R. The Language of Movement: A Guidebook to Choretics. Plymouth: Macdonald & Evans; 1974.

Laban R. The Mastery of Movement. Plymouth: Macdonald & Evans; 1988.

Laban, Lawrence FC. Effort. London: Macdonald & Evans; 1974.

Leste A, Rust J. Effects of dance on anxiety. Journal of Perceptual Motor Skills; 1984;58:767-72.

Levy FJ. Dance/Movement Therapy: A Healing Art. Reston, VA: The American Alliance for Health, Physical Education and Dance; 1988.

Levy FJ. Dance and Other Expressive Arts Therapies: When Words Are Not Enough. New York: Routledge; 1995.

Lamb W, Turner D. Management Behavior. London: Duckworth; 1969.

Lamb W. Internal Motivation: An Important Aspect of Top Team Planning. Human and Industrial Relations—A Working Handbook. Kluwer-Harrap Handbooks; 1975. pp. 2.7.1-01-2.7.1-13.

Lamb W. Movement awareness as a management aid. Personal Executive, 1981. pp. 21-4.

Lamb W, Watson E. Body Code: The Meaning in Movement. London and Boston: Routhledge & Kegan Paul; 1979.

Lunardi AC, Marques da Silva CC, Rodrigues Mendes FA, Marques AP, Stelmach R, Fernandes Carvalho CR. How to Choose between CT and MRI. Journal of Asthma. 2011;48(1):105-10.

Mehrabian A, Ferris SR. Inferences of attitudes from non-verbal communication in two channels. Journal Consult, Psychol. 1967;31:246-52.

Moore CL. Executives in Actions: A Guide to Balanced Decision-Making in Management. Plymouth: Macdonald & Evans; 1982.

North M. Personality Assessment through Movement. Boston: Plays Inc.; 1975.

Payne H. Dance Movement Therapy: Theory and Practice. New York: Tavistock/Routledge; 1992.

Porterfield JA, DeRosa C. Mechanical Neck Pain—Perspectives in Functional Anatomy. Philadelphia: WB Sunders Company; 1995.

Ramsden P, Zacharias J. Action-Profiling-generating competitive edge through realizing management potential. Vermont: Gower Press; 1993.

Sandel SL. Imagery in Dance Therapy Groups: a developmental approach. In: Sandel SL, Chaiklin S, Lohn A (Eds). Foundations of Dance/Movement Therapy: The Life and Work of Marian Chase. Columbia, MD: The Marian Chace Memorial Fund of the American Dance Therapy Association. 1993a. pp. 112-20.

Schmais C. Dance therapy in perspective. In: Mason K (Ed). Dance Therapy Focus on Dance VII. Reston, VA: American Alliance for Health, Physical Education, Recreation and Dance; 1974. pp. 7-12.

Scully R, Barnes M. Physical Therapy. J.B. East Washington Square, Philadelphia: Lippincott Company; 1989.

Shainberg C. Kabbalah and the Power of Dreaming—Awakening the Visionary Life. Lake Book Manufacturing, Inc. 2005.

Shafer K, Greenfield F. Asthma Free in 21 days. Harper San Francisco; 2000.

Wright J, Mischel W. Influence of affect on cognitive social learning person variables. Journal of Personality and Social Psychology. 1982;43:901-14.

Appendix

History and Development of Action Profiling

Around the turn of the 20th century, the standardization of mechanical parts and mass production forced scientists to begin looking at a hitherto unstudied aspect of industrialization—the physical movements of the line worker (Moore, 1982). The goal of these scientific studies was to lower production costs, raise profits and enhance the efficiency of the workers' movements. These studies were conducted by filming line workers in action, analyzing their movements and then trying to cut out any unnecessary moves.

In 1928, Laban developed a notation system which could be used to record human movements. Lawrence, a management consultant, latched onto Laban and his ideas. He began bringing Laban into the field to study workers' movements. Once in the factories, Laban switched his interest from the structural aspects of motion (which part of the body is in motion, where it moves in space, etc.) to energy usage, or effort. Laban (1988, p. 9) defined effort as "the inner impulses from which movement originates." By finding new effort rhythms for doing the work, Laban was able to train women to perform some heavy-duty jobs previously carried out by men.

After World War II, Laban continued to test his ideas on efficiency with the help of Warren Lamb. Their goal was to determine the correct effort rhythm for a particular line job, find a manager or worker with a particular aptitude who could be trained in that rhythm and then match the two up. At the beginning, the rhythm of an individual's movement on the job was notated and analyzed, then the movement profile was compared to a job description in order to predict a person's suitability to the job. Later, instead of watching a manager or worker performing the job, they could discern the suitability by way of a standard interview.

Table 1: Concave Shape-Planes-Convex Shape

Concave shape	Planes	Convex shape
Enclosing	Horizontal (table)	Spreading
Descending	Vertical (door)	Rising
Receding	Sagittal (wheel)	Advancing

In 1952, Lamb opened his own management consulting practice and developed his movement profiling techniques independently of Laban. In a process of refining his observation techniques and interpretative framework, the Aptitude Assessment was created as a profile that revealed managerial aptitude (Har-El, 1991).

WHAT IS AN ACTION-PROFILE

According to Carol-Lynne Moore (1982), Action-Profiling is an observational tool geared to help managers understand movement styles and appreciate the distinctive patterns of workers in the workplace. The Action-Profile is a systematic technique used for studying managerial and work behavior via movements, aiming to enhance personal performance and team organizational effectiveness.

According to Lamb and Watson (1979), when we move, we carry our space with us. "Our" space is the area in which we can extend our limbs and torso. This is known as our kinesphere, or the space within which we move. We can examine how movement is shaped within our own kinesphere by either carrying out simple actions, such as getting dressed, or by concentrating on a single reaching movement where posture is involved.

Our kinesphere forms a sphere or globe surrounding our body, within which all our movements extend to our own physical limits (Lamb and Watson, 1979). Movement sculptured to the physical limits involves curving, rounded, arc-like circular motions. There are various ways of moving, classified into three primary planes: (1) table (horizontal), (2) door (vertical) and (3) wheel (sagittal). These planes of motion are identified in Table 1.

History and Development of Action Profiling 153

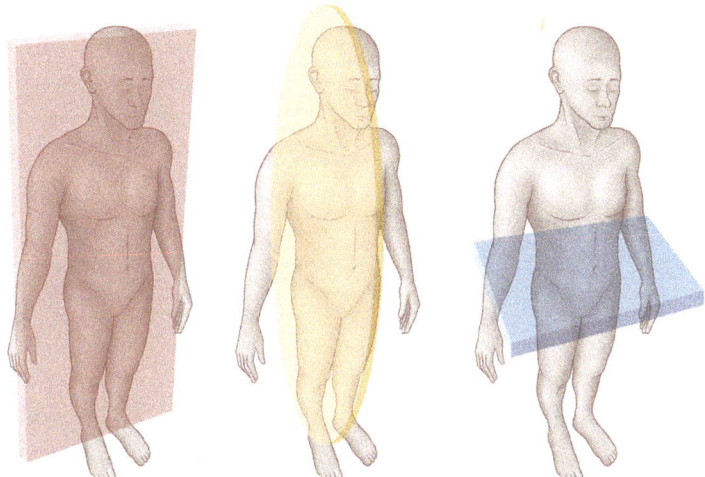

Fig. 1: Three planes of motion: Vertical (door), sagittal (wheel), and horizontal (table).

TABLE, DOOR, AND WHEEL PLANES

It is possible to shape our movement within three primary planes in a range of varying degrees (Lamb and Watson, 1979).

Moore (1982) stated that all movement produces changes in the body. Like all sculpture, the poetry of form lies in the interaction between the mass of the moving body and the empty space around it. In order to describe the sculpture of movement, we need to be able to map these shapes by creating a three-dimensional "longitude and latitude" for the kinesphere which will help us locate the spatial pathways of the body parts in motion. Moore (1982) trisected our kinesphere into three planes. These planes intersect at the center of the body and take their spatial orientation from the body. Each of these planes divides the kinesphere in half (Fig. 1). She describes:

1. The door plane slices vertically through the body from head to toe, separating the front of the body from the back. The door plane's primary dimension is height; its secondary dimension is width. It extends up and down, and to the right and left of the body.

2. The wheel plane bisects the body along its vertical axis, separating the right side from the left side. Its primary dimension is depth; its secondary dimension is height. It extends in front of and behind the body, and also upward and downward.
3. The table plane bisects the body at the waist level. Its primary dimension is width; its secondary dimension is depth. It extends to the right and left, and in front of and behind the body. It separates the head, chest, and arms from the hips and legs (Moore, 1982, p. 69).

When we observe other people's movement, we often find that people have a stronger tendency for moving in one of the three planes. For example, the vertically (door)-oriented mover seems to be segregating the front from the back of her body; therefore, when we interact with this person, we sense that her stance may be marking a territorial boundary.

Lamb and Watson (1979) described experiments with teachers and children that showed that a teacher who uses primarily vertically oriented movement will be successful in getting the children to follow the instructions: "No one is to come past me." When the same statement is made by a teacher who uses horizontally oriented movement, children perceive her attitude as more open and inviting, and they may not want to stop approaching her.

The person who tends to use the forward-backward (sagittal) orientation interacts differently with the environment on the left and right sides of her body. This movement has an ordering, organizing character. For example, a teacher in the playground who tries to divide children into different teams will achieve success more readily when predominantly using the sagittal orientation (Lamb and Watson, 1979).

North (1978) spoke about where the body action takes place in the space surrounding the body and where the shapes of the gestures are placed in relation to the body: high, across, or to the open side of the body, in front or behind. She adds that the recognition of the shapes which every person uses can give us another clue to her movement configuration. However, the configuration/action sequences occur because we initiate movement with our effort.

Table 2: Three Effort-Shape Affinities

Affinity	Shape	Affinity
Spreading	Horizontal	Enclosing
Circling	Direction Effort	Pointing
Rising	Vertical	Descending
Decreasing	Pressure Effort	Increasing
Advancing	Sagittal	Receding
Decelerating	Timing Effort	Accelerating

EFFORT-SHAPE AFFINITIES

Shape can be defined as the configuration the body makes in space. As you shape your movement within your kinesphere, you apply effort to obtain variation. You not only shape your movement in one of the three planes, but you also accompany these shapes using variations of the three effort components: (1) direction, (2) timing and (3) pressure (Lamb and Watson, 1979).

The effort components can be defined as follows:

> *Direction*: how you move through space;
> *Timing*: how quickly or slowly you complete an action;
> *Pressure*: how you use the mass of your body.

Shape and effort are the two processes by which we create movement. The relationship between them is important for our understanding of movement behavior. There is no automatic correlation between effort variation and shaping variation; in theory, any particular effort may be combined with any particular shape. However, in practice, some efforts work out best when applied to certain shapes. When you combine an effort which seems to be in harmony with the shape of your movement, you are bound to achieve effort-shape affinity.

Three effort-shape affinities have been identified: (1) horizontal shape-direction effort, (2) vertical shape-pressure effort and (3) sagittal shape-timing effort. The affinities are identified in Table 2 (Lamb and Watson, 1979).

Lamb and Watson (1979) described the insight that we can achieve watching the effort-shape affinities of the person we are observing:

"The reactions to these different combinations tell us a great deal. If affinity movements are used in the sagittal zone, then other people either get a 'come on' message from the advancing-decelerating combination, or a 'let's get ready' message from the retiring-accelerating combination. Those with similar sagittal affinity will respond positively to these messages, whereas non-affinitive movements in this plane tend to isolate the performer as though to say 'count me out!' Sadly, the silent language may convey this message through non-affinity, when the person desperately wants to be counted in. Non-affinity in movement brings frustration" (p. 80).

Moore (1982) described the distance, force and time as the mechanical factors which affect all physical movement, including the movement of our body. Human movements can be analyzed according to these factors, where the body is seen as an engine moving a set of weights and bone levers, overcoming gravity and resisting momentum. However, Moore pointed out that in Action-Profiling we are dealing with movement as a communication system and not a mechanical phenomenon. It is the quality of the movement, and not the quantity, which is of great interest to the action profiler.

Laban (1988) discussed the components making up the different effort qualities which result from an inner attitude (conscious or subconscious) toward the motion factors of weight, space, time and flow. Effort elements are also used to describe a person's style. They include: weight, time and space. Each element can be described according to two aspects. The quantitative aspects of movement are operative and objectively measurable. The qualitative aspects of movement are personal and classifiable. Weight (quantitative) consists of firm and fine touch (qualitative); time (quantitative) consists of sudden and sustained (qualitative); space (quantitative) consists of direct and flexible (qualitative) (Laban, 1988) [Table 3 (Moore, 1982)].

North (1975) distinguished between the quantitative and qualitative aspects of movement. The quantitative motion factors can be described as the amount of space, weight, time and flow. Qualitatively, the motion factors can be described as the moving person's "attitude toward" space (e.g. the flexibility or directedness of attention), weight (e.g. the sensitivity or forcefulness of intention), time (e.g. the

Table 3: Quantitative Factors-Qualitative Factors	
Quantitative factors	Qualitative factors
Distance	Varying focus Direct ⟷ Indirect
Force	Varying pressure Increasing pressure ⟷ Decreasing pressure
Time	Varying pace Accelerating ⟷ Decelerating
Tension	Varying flow Binding ⟷ Freeing

indulgence or urgency of decision), and flow (e.g. the ease or restraint of the action). The qualitative aspects of movement have special significance in personality assessment due to their potential ability to reveal the mental or emotional relationships to the movement.

Developmentally we tend to spread or enclose our body before we rise or descend. The logic of the sequence is evident in studies of children, or adults in a learning situation. For example, when young children face new situations, they go through a primary stage where they may tend to use the horizontal orientation (give attention) while staying close to a parent/adult or standing still. Then there is a stage when they begin to look as though they are planning to do something using the vertical orientation (the intention stage). Suddenly, without further warning, they are off using the sagittal orientation (acting on some decision) (Lamb and Turner, 1969).

"In all movement there must necessarily be variation in both shape and effort components, though the amount of variation in the respective categories may differ considerably. Some people appear to be making great efforts over a wide range while retaining more or less the same shape. Others vary the shape a lot but repeat a similar effort over and over again" (Lamb and Turner, 1969, p. 67).

FOUR EFFORT-SHAPE QUALITATIVE FACTORS AMONG SENIOR MANAGERS

Although human body movement is governed by factors of distance, force and time, the human being has the power to vary these factors qualitatively. Moore (1982) described four qualitative factors of movement which were discovered through direct observation of the behavior of senior managers:

1. The varying *focus* provides a means of orienting oneself physically or emotionally in a straightforward, direct way, or in a flexible, indirect way.

   "The readiness to vary focus in integrated whole-body action reveals an investigative management style. The investigative manager is characteristically curious, inquisitive and analytical, and this felt sense is expressed physically by variations in focus. The investigative manager directs, probing for information, scanning and categorizing data. This physical tendency to orientate oneself by changing focus reveals a need to act in an investigative manner," (Moore, 1982, p. 60).

2. Variations in *pressure* add to the range of what a person can do with her actual weight and muscular strength. The meaning of pressure variation, as described by Moore (1982) is:

   "The readiness to vary pressure in integrated whole-body action reveals a determined management style. The determined manager is characteristically resolute and purposeful, and this felt sense is expressed physically in variations in pressure. The physical tendency to exert pressure in varying degrees to convince oneself or persuade others, reveals a need to act in a determined manner," (p. 62).

3. *Pace* is the process of changing tempo, of accelerating or decelerating the speed of a motion. It deals with noticeable variations in speed. The meaning of pace variations as described by Moore (1982) is:

   "The ability to vary pace in integrated whole-body actions reveals a time-keeping management style. The time-keeping manager is a go-getter, prompt, methodical, competitive, and this felt sense is expressed physically by variations in pace. The time-keeper controls the pacing of implementation; he speeds up and slows down action in order to move at the most appropriate moment. This physical tendency to alter the pacing of commitment reveals a need to act in a time-keeping manner," (p. 64).

4. All movement produces *muscular tension*; a muscle works by contracting (tensing) and exerting a pull on the bony lever to which it is attached (Moore, 1982). The term "flow" was coined by Laban to describe the variations in the relationship between tensed muscles. Laban (1988) explained that the flow of movement is strongly influenced by the order in which the parts of the body are set in motion. Laban distinguished between an unhampered or "free flow" and a hampered or "bound flow."

The greatest variation in flow can be seen in the integrated whole-body actions of children. They often alternate between the freeing and binding of flow. They allow themselves to move freely and change their body flow spontaneously.

The quantitative factors of distance, force, time and tension correspond to certain qualitative factors, which are relevant to action-profiling. These kinetic qualities reveal particular kinds of action motivation: the varying *focus* (dynamic quality) correlates with the *investigatory style* (action motivation). The varying *pressure* (dynamic quality) correlates with the *determined style* (action motivation). The varying *pace* (dynamic quality) correlates with the *time-keeping style* (action motivation). The varying *flow* (dynamic quality) correlates with the intensity of need to identify oneself with activities in the work environment (action motivation).

CONNECTION BETWEEN EFFORT-SHAPE ACTIONS AND THE DECISION MAKING PROCESS

Lamb (1981) wrote about our bodies, as well as our minds, which are constantly engaged in some sort of decision-making process on different levels and at different time spans. He uses a person standing near a cliff to offer a good model of the three-stage theory of action: (1) attention, (2) intention and (3) commitment. For example, assuming that there is an "attractive object" at the foot of the cliff, we first become interested when someone mentions this to us. Our *attention* will or will not be evident, but we may be aware of a new form of body tension as we move toward developing an *intention* to investigate the "attractive object" (which we cannot see due to our distance from the edge of the cliff). When we move closer to the edge of the cliff, we recognize that the "attractive object" is a shark.

At this time we are at a point of no return, where our body tension is registered as that of *commitment* to take action. Such a process of movement from attention to intention to commitment can actually be observed in a person's body tension.

No action can be initiated without the direction of attention. Attention must be given in a particular direction as an indispensable first stage. There must be intention to act; otherwise the attention fades into passivity. Lastly, there must be a commitment to act arising from the intention. If any one of these stages is missing, action does not arise (Lamb and Watson, 1979).

Moore (1982) defined style as the way in which something is done. Style is the manner and means by which action is executed. Management style, then, is how an individual goes about making a decision. To better understand the relationship of style and action, it is helpful to visualize decision-making in the three stage process: (1) attention, (2) intention and (3) commitment.

Attention: The first stage in decision-making involves getting oriented to the problem, which needs to be resolved. The activities which take place in this stage include probing, questioning old assumptions, seeking alternatives, breaking assumptions, etc. This stage includes the preliminary research and survey necessary before a decision can be made.

Intention: In the second stage a course of action must be determined. The purpose of the proposed action is clarified and a firm resolution is established. Unless the resolution to act is established and strongly supported, interest fades and there will be no action. Thus, this stage is the critical bridge between preliminary consideration and actual execution.

Commitment: In the commitment stage the executor is convinced that she is on the right track and proceeds to implement the decision. This stage involves acting at the appropriate moment, being able to update or alter implementation, etc. The commitment stage is the stage of the process where most risks are taken. It is also often difficult or impossible to slow down or reverse direction.

SIX BASIC MANAGERIAL STYLES

Every manager attends, intends and commits on the job, yet goes about these activities in an individual manner. This is the essence of style.

Table 4: Six Basic Management Styles

Attention stage (shaping in the table plane)	
Investigative style: Probing, scanning and classifying information within a prescribed area. *Outcome*: Systematic research, establishing methods and defining standards.	*Exploratory style*: Broadening scope, uncovering, encompassing and perceiving information from many areas. *Outcome*: Creative brainstorming, discovering alternatives.
Intention stage (shaping in the door plane)	
Determined style: Affirming purpose, building resolve, forging conviction, justifying intent. *Outcome*: Persisting against odds, maintaining strength of will.	*Evaluative style*: Gauging pros and cons, analyzing the issues, perceiving proportion. *Outcome*: Clarifying intentions, realistically appraising facts and proposals.
Commitment stage (shaping in the wheel plane)	
Time-keeping: Pacing implementation, sensing the moment-by-moment timing of action. *Outcome*: Adjusting time priorities for opportune implementation.	*Anticipatory style*: Perceiving the developing stages of action and sensing the consequences of each stage. *Outcome*: Setting goals, measuring and updating plans.

Moore (1982) distinguished two different yet complimentary approaches in each of these stages. In the attention stage there are two approaches: (1) investigative and (2) exploratory. In the intention stage there are two approaches: (1) determined and (2) evaluative. In the commitment stage there are two approaches: (1) time-keeping and (2) anticipatory. The six basic management styles are outlined in Table 4 (Moore, 1982).

Moore used the three-stage action process of attention-intention-commitment to depict six basic management styles. The investigative, determined and time-keeping styles have to do with the exertion of particular kinds of mental and physical energies. These managers work through focus, pushing and pacing their action to make things happen. They are assertive and apply effort in their approach. On the other hand, the exploratory, evaluative and anticipatory styles are concerned with relating decisions to each other on the whole. These managers are concerned with getting perspective on their decisions. They are less assertive than investigators, determiners and time-keepers. They design their decisions to achieve the desired results rather than pushing for action.

ACTION-PROFILING AND THE INDIVIDUAL STYLE

The Action-Profiling technique can be used to discern the following aspects of personal style: which stages of the decision-making process an executive prefers; whether she is inclined to take a more assertive or perceptive approach; how adaptable she is; and how intense her need to identify is. According to Moore (1982), senior managers will restyle their jobs to suit their personal action preferences. For instance, an intention-oriented manger will focus on policy-making and difficult projects, which test his convictions.

In general, Action-Profiling accommodates the individual style. It enables an individual to understand her decision-making style and to use this understanding in order to develop effective work tools as well as good relationships with coworkers.

DRAWING A PROFILE

Lamb (1975) identified how an individual could draw a personal profile by following interview and counseling sessions with an Action-Profile consultant. The percentage shown in the action profiles represents the relative amount of time and energy which the individual allots to every aspect of decision-making. In practice it takes about 20-30 minutes to make an observation. The conclusions are expressed in words and the capacities are tabulated for purposes of comparison.

Moore (1982) used an example of Mr J.F. Gary, a chief executive of a medium-sized company that manufactures industrial goods. At the time his profile was drawn, Mr. Gary had been in his job less than six months. His Action-Profile report is depicted in Table 5 (Moore, 1982).

Lamb and Watson (1979) suggested drawing up an Action-Profile by first listing the three stages of action and filling in beside each a percentage allocation of the action energy which matches the movement. Then divide each of these action stages into the

Table 5: The Action-Profile Report	
Attention (Table plane)	
Investigating	23%
Exploring	6%
Intention (Door plane)	
Determining	6%
Evaluating	22%
Commitment (Wheel plane)	
Timing	29%
Anticipating	14%

assertion-perspective states in which they are expressed, and subdivide the percentage allocations. The last step entails the evaluation of the most important features, which will lead to the drawing of the conclusions. When a profile is made, the interviewer attempts to discover the movement patterns which will reveal the unique action motivation of the manager being interviewed. The complexity of these movement patterns varies from person to person. Some patterns are obvious while others are subtle or elusive and require extensive and careful observation before they can be pinpointed.

Index

Page numbers followed by *f* and *t* refer to figures and tables respectively.

A

Abdominal cavity 22
Action-profile assessment 7
Action-profile consultant 162
Action-profile report 163*t*
   attention (table plane) 163*t*
      exploring 163*t*
      investigating 163*t*
   commitment (wheel plane) 163*t*
      anticipating 163*t*
      timing 163*t*
   intention (door plane) 163*t*
      determining 163*t*
      evaluating 163*t*
Action-profiling and the individual style 162
Action profiling theory 4
Aerobic training 1
Alexander technique 12
Analysis of the test 3
Analyzing the patient's responses 141
Architectural metaphor 145
Asthma 4
Asthma attacks 87

B

Balanced movement pattern 51
Balanced usage of direct and indirect movements 51
Base of diaphragmatic muscle 97
Basic management styles 161*t*
   attention stage (shaping in the table plane) 161*t*
      exploratory style 161*t*
      investigative style 161*t*
   commitment stage (shaping in the wheel plane) 161*t*
      anticipatory style 161*t*
      time-keeping 161*t*
   intention stage (shaping in the door plane) 161*t*
      determined style 161*t*
      evaluative style 161*t*
Basic principles of RiVision 17
Benefits of RiVision 1
Betty's body awareness 76
Betty's imaginative roots 75*f*
Betty's range of motion 74
Blue vase 99
Body misalignment 7
Body movement style 3
Body's physical limits 30
Body-tuning 11
Bonsai tree 79
Bound flow 51
Breathing exercises 12
Breathing pattern 22

C

Cathartic nature of dance 1
Cervical and thoracic spine 87

Cervical range of motion (CROM) 1
Chace technique 13
Chronic neck pain 1, 4
Chronic pain 2
Chronic pain sufferers 5
Chronic physical and emotional pain 4
Complementary therapies 2
Components of RiVision 11
Connection between effort-shape actions and the decision making process 159
Continuum ranging 40
Conventional physical therapy 103
Conventional physical therapy treatment 2

D

Dance/Movement therapy (DMT) 1, 13
   Chace technique 13
   guided imagery 14
Determined style 159
Direct movement 46
Door plane 8
Dynamic quality 159

E

Effects of DMT on mood 1
Effort-shape affinities 155
Elliptical balloon 98
Emotional experience 30
Emotional factors 2
Expansion of motion 17
Experience of hostile environment 140*t*
Experience of pleasant environment 142*t*

F

Feldenkrais technique 12
Five motion factors of RiVision 20
   awareness 20
   grounding 20
   muscle tension 20

   orienting 20
   pacing 20
Forward-backward orientation 154
Free/Bound flow scale 52
Free flow 51
Free flow (soft) versus bound flow (rigid) movement patterns 55
Frustration issue 14

G

Gestures or body posture 28
Goal of the Chace technique 146
Golden shield 112
Graceful blade of grass 53
Greater range of motion 19
Grounding exercise 38
Groundwork for RiVision 21
Guided imagery 5, 35
Guide to Betty's treatment 66
   encounter I 66
      goal 66
         body awareness exercises 66
         guided imagery 66
   encounter II 69
      goal 69
         guided imagery 69
   encounter III 70
      goal 71
         guided imagery 71
   encounter IV 72
      goal 74
         guided imagery 74
         physical exercises 76
   encounter V 78
      goal 78
         dance/movement therapy 78
         guided imagery 79
   encounter VI 81
      goal 81
         dance/movement therapy 83
         guided imagery 82
   encounter VII 84
      goal 84
         dance/movement therapy 84

Guide to Cha's treatment 103
   encounter I 103
      goal 104, 107
         combining dance/movement
            therapy and guided
            imagery 108
         guided imagery 104
   encounter II 108
      goal 109
         dance/movement therapy 110
   encounter III 112
      goal 112
         dance/movement therapy 114
         guided imagery 112
   encounter IV 115
      goal 115
         dance/movement therapy and
            guided imagery 115
         guided imagery 115
   encounter V 116
   encounter VI 117
      goal 118
         guided imagery 118
   encounter VII 120
      goal 120
         body awareness exercises 120
         guided imagery 121
Guide to Jane's treatment 124
   encounter I 124
      goal 124
         body awareness exercises 125
   encounter II 130
      goal 130
         body awareness exercises 130
         breathing exercises 131
   encounter III 132
      goal 132
         body awareness and physical
            exercises 133
         body awareness exercises 133
Guide to Wen's treatment 88
   encounter I 88
      goal 88
         guided imagery 88
   encounter II 91
      goal 91
         guided imagery 91

   encounter III 93
      goal 95
         body awareness and dance/
            movement therapy 95
         guided imagery 95
   encounter IV 97
      goal 99
         guided imagery 99
   encounter V 101
      goal 101
         breathing exercises 101

H

Holistic approach combining 78
Home program regimen 19
Horizontal plane 3
Hostile environment 139
Human motion 8
Human movements 156

I

Idiosyncratic patterns 145
Imaginative roots exercise 36
Imaginative shield 112
Increased muscle spasm 87
Indirect movement 46
Indirect movement quality 46
Inside-body experience 30
Integrated forms of therapy 2
Investigatory style 159

J

Joint mobilization 11

K

Kinetic qualities 159

L

Level of self-esteem 3
Lower back pain 2
Lubrication 53

M

Massage and therapeutic exercises 3
Mood adjective checklist 15
Motion factors 4
Movement behavior 13
Movement pace 46
Movement profile 151
Movement sensation 33
Multidimensional treatment 137
Muscle activity 7
Muscle tension 7
Muscle tension exercise 55
Muscular tension 51
Musculoskeletal disorders 2, 8
Musculoskeletal dysfunction 7
Musculoskeletal injuries 1
Myofascial release 11

N

Neck exercises 1
Normal flux 51
Normal gait pattern 28

O

Orienting exercise 48
Orienting movement quality 46
Outside-body experience 30

P

Pacing exercise 42
Part of RiVision 8
Patterns of movement 32, 33
Pendulum 100
Personal profile 162
Physical sensation 2, 20
Physical therapy 1, 11
   breathing exercises 12
   functional approaches 12
      Alexander technique 12
      Feldenkrais technique 12
   hands-on techniques 11
      body tuning 11
      joint mobilization 11
      myofascial release 11
      soft tissue mobilization 11
   therapeutic exercises 12
Physical treatment 74
Pleasant environment 139
Powerful relaxation technique 12
Pressure motion quality 40
Principles of RiVision 5
Protective shield 116
Psychological benefits 3

Q

Qualitative factors 157*t*
Quality of the motion 53
Quality of the movement 33, 49, 51
Quantitative and qualitative aspects of movement 156
Quantitative factors 157*t*, 159

R

Repetitive stress injury 137
Repetitive stress pattern 137
Rhythmic movement relationship 14
Rib cage area 87
Rib cage musculature 87
RiVision method 1

S

Sagittal plane 3
Severe pain maneuver 40
Shoulder pain 65
Social participation 3
Soft tissue inflammation 11
Specific cause-effect formula 57
Sternum bone 87
Symbolism in DMT 14

T

Tailoring RiVision 18
Tension in the musculature of the back 9

Theoretical foundation of dance therapy 13
Therapeutic movement relationship 14
Three planes of motion 9
  horizontal (table) 9*f*
  sagittal (wheel) 9*f*
  vertical (door) 9*f*
Tightness and spasm of the soft tissue 7
Torso and extremities 41
Torso region 26
Traditional physical therapy approach 3
Treatment protocols 12
Treatment protocols in RiVision 18
  combined therapies 18
    combination of DMT and guided imagery 18
    combination of physical therapy and DMT 18
    combination of physical therapy and guided imagery 18
    combination of physical therapy, DMT and guided imagery 18
  single therapies 18
    dance/movement therapy (DMT) 18
    guided imagery 18
    physical therapy 18
Treatment solutions 3

U

Usage of DMT and guided imagery 146

V

Vertical plane 3

W

Wave-like movement 76
Wen's chest area 87
Wen's inefficient breathing pattern 101
Wen's posture and breathing habits 87
Wheel plane 8

www.ingramcontent.com/pod-product-compliance
Lightning Source LLC
Chambersburg PA
CBHW040516220526
45473CB00012B/2882